Laughter, Learning and Gratitude

on a Journey with Alzheimer's

MARLENE LONEY

About the Book

This is a book about Alzheimer's that is funny, positive and heartfelt. The author Marlene Loney documented the twelve year journey with her mother in short stories and ultimately reframed the tragedy of Alzheimer's into a positive life changing experience. Flip to any page and find a short story that is applicable to the journey. Offering readers insights and encouragement and community along with the unexpected benefits of giving care. This book celebrates the life of her mother and shares what the disease taught her about her capacity to love.

Laughter, Learning, and Gratitude on a Journey with Alzheimer's reframes the pervasive narrative surrounding Alzheimer's, one filled with pain and suffering, to one of positivity and dignity. This isn't to say that it's easy—far from it. But caregivers can find humour, even if it's twisted, and joy in the smallest moments. These anecdotes are filled with practical information and survival strategies for caregivers. Yes, survival strategies, because as Marlene shares with vulnerability and grace, when we care for others, we often stop caring for ourselves.

Laughter, Learning, and Gratitude on a Journey with Alzheimer's is more than a memoir; it's a celebration of love that asks us to do what's best for our loved ones and ultimately ourselves.

More comments from the professionals...

"Losing my 49 year old niece to frontal-temporal dementia tuned me into the poignancy of this story and the very honest way that Marlene relates it. This is a story well worth reading and then referring to others."
—Michael M Myckatyn MD, President, Minoru Medical Education Society

"Insightful, poignant, funny and sad as well as helpful for others who find themselves in the same situation."
—Michael Frey MD, UBC Clinical Assistant Professor, Dept. Family Practice

"This book brings you right into the unscripted realities of life as a caregiver. It is both heartwarming and sad as the reflections speak the truth. Recommended reading for any health care provider working with older adults including nursing and personal support worker students to improve understanding and develop empathy for the lived experiences."
—Kerilynn Bath, Registered Nurse and College Educator

"This book helps lessen the fear and ease the burden of the journey. Marlene offers examples of how she learned to appreciate the good times, even during the difficult stages of the diseases' progression, and reminds us that we are not alone in this journey."
—Catherine Butler, Professional Care Aid and Team Member

◆ FriesenPress

One Printers Way
Altona, MB R0G 0B0
Canada

www.friesenpress.com

ISBN
978-1-03-831029-3 (Hardcover)
978-1-03-831028-6 (Paperback)
978-1-03-831030-9 (eBook)

1. BIOGRAPHY & AUTOBIOGRAPHY, PERSONAL MEMOIRS

Distributed to the trade by The Ingram Book Company

Dedication

This book is dedicated to all who venture on the path of caregiving. My heart goes out to those who face challenges much greater than mine under more adverse conditions. All we can do is our best and it will be enough.

Proceeds from the sale of this book will go towards the support of caregivers.

Table of Contents

Every Moment Counts— Introduction

This book is intended to reframe the tragedy of Alzheimer's in a positive light. Not easy and sometimes twisted with lots of humour and grace. A place where caregivers will find laughter and positive insights.

What you will find in these pages is funny stories and moments of learning with positive outcomes, which for me was the whole damn journey, in the end. Never mind the moments of complete and utter despair or the times when my body was shaking with anger and frustration. Reframe and focus on the positive—always! The stories are sorted by disease progression on a loose timeline, but flip to any page and you will find a short story that is applicable to the journey.

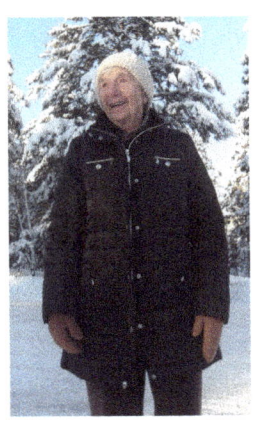

Mom's face always lit up when outdoors.

All the stories are about the unexpected benefits of giving care, of how we grow when given the rare opportunity to love in this way, and how this challenge makes us better people. My mother taught me so much in the last years of her life that I will be forever grateful for the opportunity I was given.

Without Alzheimer's, I would never have received these lessons in love and capacity. This book is my way of sharing the positive life-changing moments that make caring an opportunity not to be missed at whatever level you can individually manage. I was "all in" as my dear friend said and have no regrets.

Ultimately, this book's intent is to celebrate the life of my mother and what the disease taught me about my capacity to serve, care, and love. I hope to encourage others already on this journey and to motivate others to walk down this road.

I started with a blog and Facebook page during COVID-19. Most of what is written here you will also find if you search for "Alzheimer's Blog Forum Canada." I often flooded new caregivers with information and thought if I started a blog, perhaps I could help just one person on this journey. The book's intent is the same.

Hopefully, those that are wrapped up deeply in this drama will have a moment to read and be helped. My heart goes out to everyone making tough decisions and doing more than they ever thought possible. I am a bit afraid of what you will think of my writing, but I am also excited to help just one person on this road. Join me in finding the positive!

Sincerely,
Marlene Loney MD (Mother's Daughter)

The Early Years Lost

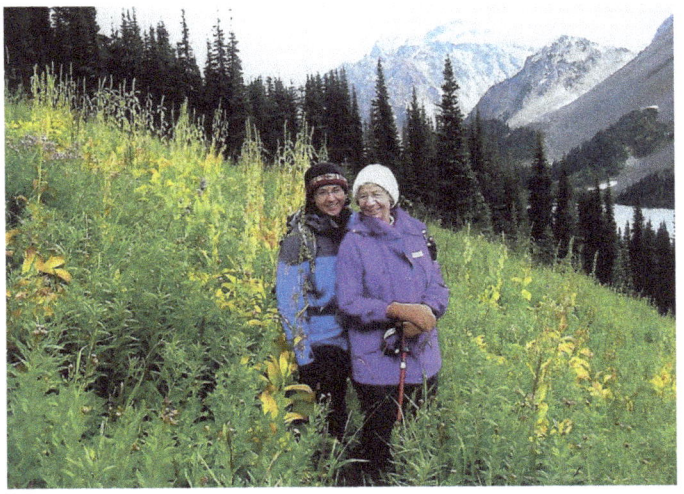

Fall hiking trip in the Whistler area.

I am grateful that I did not run from this disease and took the opportunity to do things with Mom while she still could. Memories of our two big hiking trips will always be with me. If my mom had not been diagnosed, I never would have made the time to do things with her. One day, I would have received a call that my busy, healthy mom was gone and would grieve what could have been. Alzheimer's forced me to *do it NOW!*

When Mom was first diagnosed, we had gone for a hike in the hills close to home. We were sitting on a rock enjoying the view and contemplating the future. Mom had always been interested in Eastern religions, and I said that now more than ever she would be living in the moment. Savouring each sunrise for the first time. I was still fighting the diagnosis and hoped it was wrong, but the only way to get a definitive diagnosis was a brain autopsy. We both agreed that was a drastic measure for the peace of mind that certainty brings and passed on the procedure.

Of course, that early conversation filled with laughter did not prepare my mother for the moment when she knew I was her child but had no recollection of me as an infant. How can you forget your baby? We had gone on our second big hiking trip when that hit her. For an entire night, we cried together and held each other close as I tried to give her, through my love, a sense that I was hers. Her despair over this loss was gut-wrenching. Fortunately, she also forgot what she forgot, so with time, the disease was kinder.

Packing for Mom

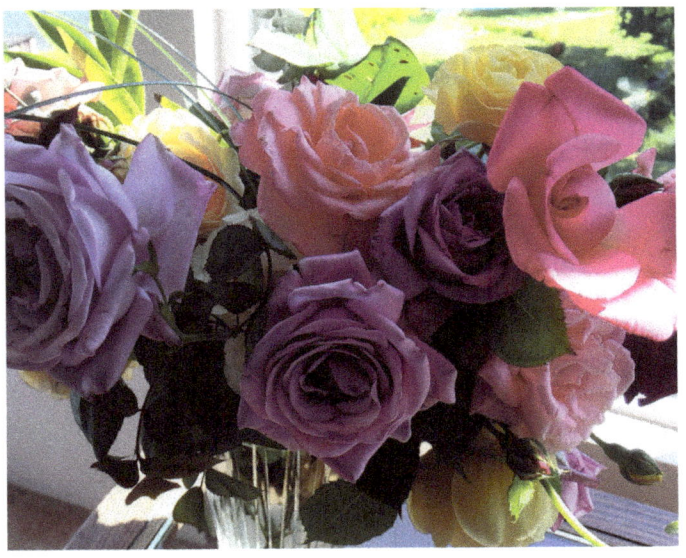

Flowers from a team member's garden.

Mom and I had to go to Vancouver to visit the Alzheimer's clinic at UBC. After the appointment, I thought to make the trip a bit more fun we would travel on to Victoria for the spring flowers. Packing was no longer easy for Mom, so we did it together. She watched as I confidently packed a bag. A chore she had done countless times for me when I was a child. No worries, Mom. I got this!

On arrival in Victoria, I had booked a charming B and B where the first floor was actually the second floor up a steep flight of steps! Good job, Marlene! Mom steadied herself and tackled the stairs with a deep breath.

We both slept quite well, and after showering, we were ready to dress for the day. Mom: "Did you pack undies for me?" Oh, crap! I had forgotten that one item of clothing. So much for being the expert. I still needed my mother to remind me to pack clean underwear. "No worries, Mom. Use a pair of mine. They are stretchy, and we can shop for you today." The image of my undies halfway up her hips and the two of us howling with laughter will be forever with me.

Thank you, Mom, for all the great memories you have given me.

Letting Go of YOUR Social Anxieties

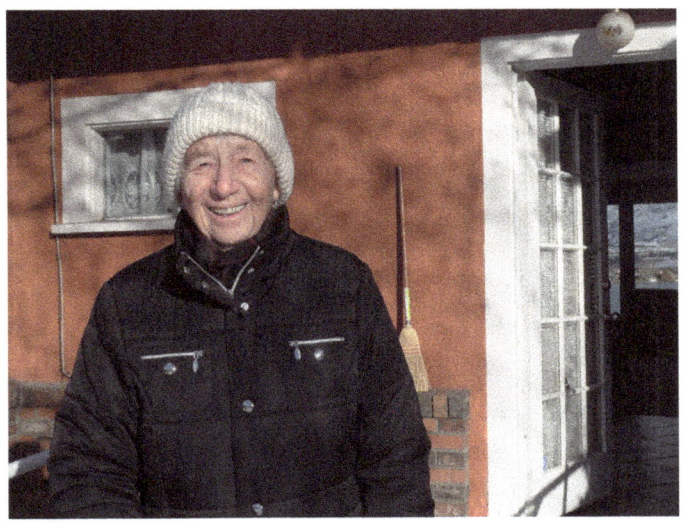

Who could resist that smile?

Mom was always friendly and warm and willing to give the best hugs. Along with her brain having a best before date that was long past, so were her arteries well past their best days. She had almost lost her foot to artery disease a few years previous, and we were on our way back to Kelowna for a follow-up appointment. I learned to plan slowly and was running a bit late. Making good time, I took advantage of the passing lane up a hill and passed a bunch of cars—and on the crest of the hill was immediately pulled over by the police." Licence please, ma'am. Do you know how fast you were going?" Sheesh . . . I am looking after my mother! Can't he see my angel wings! What is this harassment! He handed me a ticket for $120. "Drive safe, take it slower, have a nice day." As we pulled back into the heavy traffic, even later than before, Mom reframed it for me: "He seems like a nice man!" Sheesh!!!

The doctor's appointment did not go well, and we ended up having to stay the night. That evening, we were slowly walking along the waterfront, enjoying the breeze. A man in his late forties was leaning on his bicycle near a patio bar. He was smiling. Mom gravitated to his smile and returned it with one of hers. "You look like someone I know," she said, and moments later, I found the three of us in a warm embrace. He was a total stranger and simply accepted my mom's hug. I was uncomfortable at first, this was my mother who lacked proper social boundaries, and then I just rolled with the moment. Everyone needs hugs! Perhaps we should all let go of some of our social boundaries.

As we left this happy, pleasant man, we came across two ladies sitting on a bench. Mom smiled warmly, and I could see them stiffen and shy away from her. New wrinkles forming instantly on their scrunched faces. We seem to want to hide our elderly and demented away as though their disease is contagious. Mom's only crime was being too friendly.

In Calgary, this past November as I was putting a few boxes in the garage, just across the lane a homeless man was looking in garbage cans for bottles. I called him over to give him a big bag of change that was rattling around in my purse. "It looks like you are having a rough time. Here, these are for you." He said, "Hey, thanks. Would you like a hug?" And suddenly I found myself caught up in his warm and friendly embrace. It made me think of my mother and the lesson I had learned.

Travel, Friends, and UBC

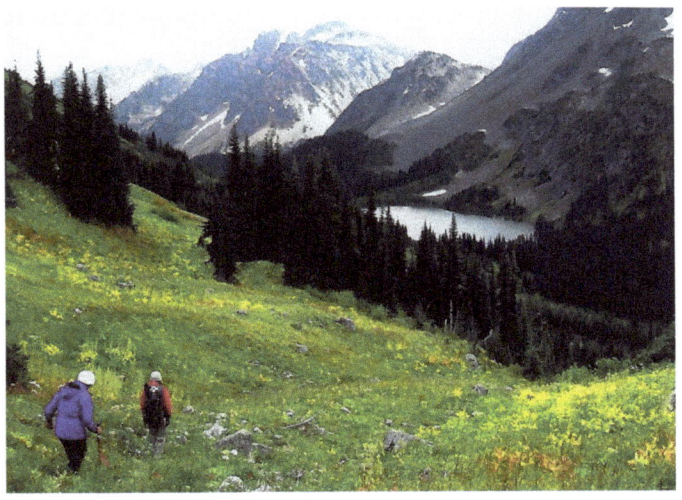

One of our last big hikes together.

This trip to UBC went much better. There was no great news from the good doctor but involving Mom with UBC gave me telephone access later in her disease for some of the decisions I had to make for her. I would speak with her local GP, the local pharmacist, and then call UBC to discuss the care plan I would be implementing. I am forever grateful for their long-distance accessibility.

We took a city bus clear across Vancouver to the base of Grouse Mountain. Mom chatted with various people on the bus, and I learned how to be less afraid of people's reactions. We took the gondola to the top, and Mom breathed in the fresh mountain air. Mountains were always home for her soul, and she beamed the entire day.

Later that evening, we met family for dinner in a local restaurant. Mom was starting to have trouble eating but still liked to go out. It was a bit tough on us as we were raised with proper table manners. I learned over time it was better to choose a spot where fewer people could watch Mom and she faced me. Easier for both of us.

She continued to enjoy restaurants for many more years and, again, was teaching other people to get over their discomfort. People would stop at our table and engage Mom in conversations as if she was the Queen!

It was interesting how many people would make the effort to chat with Mom and how charming and patient they were. On one trip, we had enjoyed a busker outside and had gone in to warm up with a coffee. When the musician came in on his break, he made a directly line to Mom to chat with her for a few minutes. She beamed with the attention and the fact that he was quite hand-some was not lost on her!

It was hard and embarrassing for me to see the change in Mom. So much had been lost. But complete strangers saw a clearly happy and well-cared-for woman who still had much to offer with just the warmth of her personality.

Building New Relationships

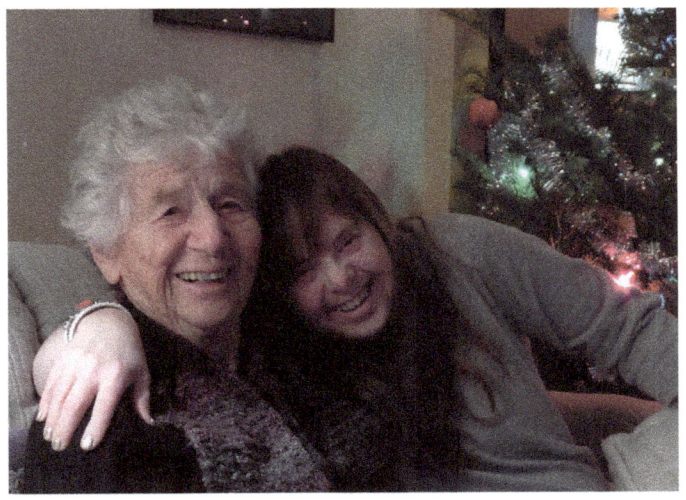

Mom with my sister.

Nothing was the same. Mom was not Mom anymore but she was still Mom. Okay, I am confused by that statement. How did my sister manage?

My sister has Down syndrome and struggled with losing her mom. But even though it was scary and sad, she persisted and a new normal was possible. Every week, one of the care team would bring Mom up to visit my sister or my sister would come down to Mom's for a visit. Many times, Mom did not seem clear that this was her youngest daughter. Sometimes, my sister would bridle with frustration but over time, I saw her also grow and care for Mom in this new situation. Gently stroking her hair and telling her to take care of herself.

My sister became one of the team and was also a source of inspiration to the other team members. It is not necessary to shelter family and friends from Alzheimer's. The disease is not contagious. She helped us see that we can all grow and change and embrace the difficult and find laughter and hope on the other side. Now when we are together, she often says, "I miss Mom" and I reply, "So do I."

My Journey

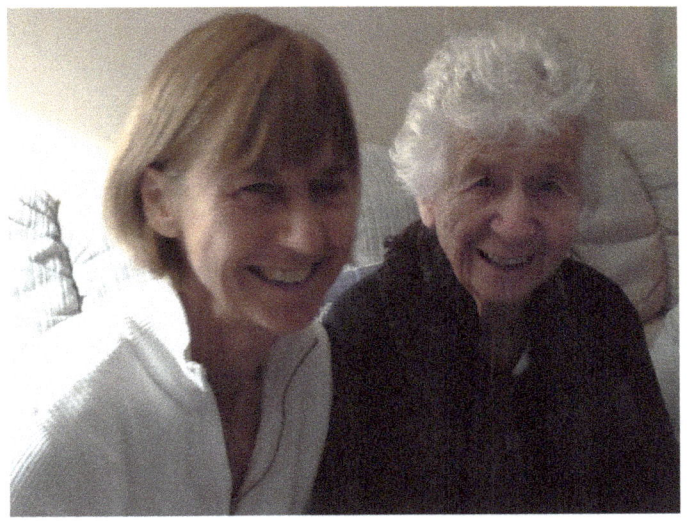

Mom and me. I see the likeness.

The question is simple: Would you do this journey if you did not have any family, if this responsibility was solely yours? My answer was YES, and I needed to accept and move on.

This was ultimately my journey, and I am stronger, more compassionate and the winner. No regrets. I call it a journey as I love to adventure travel which is about experiencing new situations and challenges that make me grow. My journey with Mom and Alzheimer's did all of that in spades.

I tried to leave space for family members to be involved and from time to time they would get on board. My story includes my father who was trying inadequately to care for my mother. My brother who never blocked any of my decisions for which I am grateful. And my Down syndrome sister who over time developed a beautiful, new relationship with Mom. Was I angry? YES. Was I sad? YES. Did my dad agree with everything I did for Mom before he passed? YES. Are my brother and I still close? YES. Am I impressed by my sister? YES!

My word for this part is "accept." I needed to move forward with conviction and do what I believed was right. This was my journey.

Nothing Happened!
Wandering Worries

Being the primary caregiver and living six hours away had its own set of frustrations. I usually woke thinking, always thinking, about solving a problem for Mom. I would get the phone calls that would roll my stomach and I would remind myself, *Nothing happened*. And that was the truth.

Mom had wandered down the road about a kilometer to a local hotel. At that stage, someone noticed her and that she seemed confused. They called the police and the police brought her home. Oh my word. That could be a cause for crisis intervention! For a family meeting!! For locking Mom away!!! But nothing happened. Mom's favourite saying was: "So

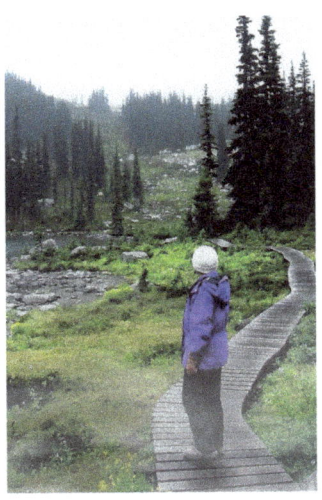

Mom on a hiking trail inhaling the fresh air and beauty.

long as you are alive LIVE." Whenever she wandered, I would clutch that saying to my heart like a mantra, wrap it around myself like a blanket. If something bad did happen, I would cry and howl and feel guilt down to my big toe, BUT I had allowed Mom to live as opposed to being locked away and safe. And nothing bad happened.

I also did what I could do to mitigate the risk. The first step was to get her a medical bracelet with her name and phone number, with her condition listed as "memory loss." I had the chain changed to something very pretty and comfortable and she never minded wearing it. Mom lived in a small town so I also registered her with the local police. I made laminated wallet cards with her name, address, and condition, and stuck them in every pocket. We put a bell on the front door that would chime whenever it was opened and this could be switched to a full alarm at night.

I also researched more complex solutions like foot insoles with trackers and bracelets with trackers. Fortunately, Mom did not wander often. Statistically, the likelihood of wandering is very high, but most Alzheimer's patients are moved towards the end of their lives and they are just trying to get back home. Leaving Mom in the home she had lived in for almost fifty years helped greatly. Oh sure, Mom at times did not remember her home and one time she looked at her husband of fifty years who was changing a light bulb and asked, "Do you work here?" It was one of my father's better days, so he kindly answered, "Yeah, sometimes."

Eating Challenges

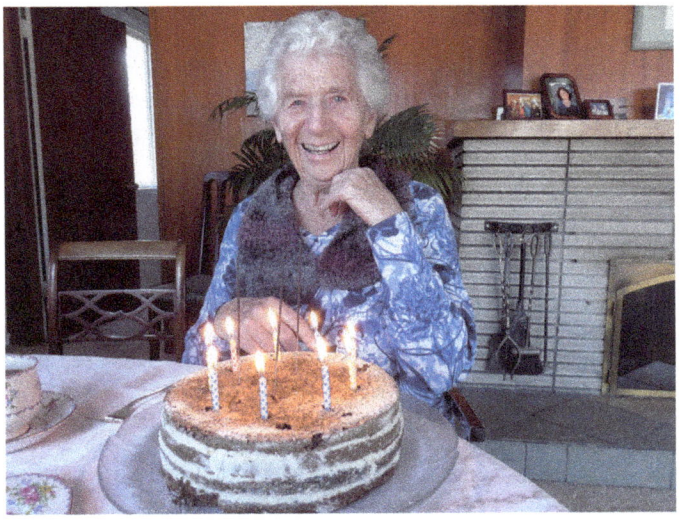

Mom enjoying a birthday celebration.

Eating changes were among the first to be noticed. Mom could not tell the size of a piece she had cut and would try and stick a huge piece of chicken in her mouth all at once. For someone that drilled us with table manners, this was a big change.

But it was also an easy fix. We would cut her food into the right-size piece. Then we found a fork and spoon with a better grip, a plate with a lip that helped keep food on the utensils, a plate with a rubber bottom that did not slide. Most of these items we found in a specialty medical equipment store or searching online for adaptive utensils.

These changes were hard for my dad to see, but he was stubborn about changing his routine. Mom and he would eat together regardless of the changes. We found colourful aprons and bibs for adults. We served finger foods as that was easy for her to manage. And we still took her out to restaurants and coffee houses.

Mom liked to set the table, but it was a random installation of art with cutlery and plates all over the clock face. She still tried to wash and dry dishes. After she was done, when she was not looking, we would put the dishes in the dishwasher for a second cleaning. I would call her efforts "the prewash."

The kitchen had always been Mom's domain and seeing others work there without her was difficult. At first, we would do it all for her until I finally understood that this was not what she wanted. We were taking over, not helping out.

Long into the disease, I would have her mixing batter and even stirring the pot, carefully watching that she did not put her hand on the element. She was still contributing and doing her job. Her mantra rings in my ears: "So long as you are alive, LIVE!"

Note to My Friends

There is something strange about Osoyoos
One meets a lot of nice people, has
them over for coffee or a meal,
They look over your books (which are
well marked with name & Tel # &
Request to please Return. and then you
never hear from them again not
even via telephone. NOTHING. for the
last 40 years,

 NOW I am out of books and FRiends !

Mom's scribbled note.

Mom passed several years ago, and this spring I finally cleaned the last few boxes that I had taken from her home. I had looked at the boxes over the past years but was always too afraid of what emotional bombs I would find. There was only one.

"There is something strange about Osoyoos. One meets a lot of nice people, has them over for a coffee or a meal. They look at your books, (which are clearly marked with name and telephone # and a request to please return) and then you never hear from them again, not even via telephone. Nothing for the last 40 years. Now I am out of books and Friends!"

I considered if I would share this story as what was positive about it, what was funny, what was the lesson to share? It just hurt to know Mom felt this way. But then I thought if this one post was read to others that are afraid of Alzheimer's, maybe, just maybe they will visit an old friend. That they will return the books, share a cup of tea, and tell stories of the times they remember. That they won't ask, "Do you know who I am?" as it is not about them. And they will give a little comfort. And while it will be hard and sad for them, their hearts will grow for doing the right thing. They will learn the disease with the disease is something they can handle and that Alzheimer's is not contagious. And maybe they will visit next week as well.

I read *Still Alice* by Lisa Genova while Mom was in an early stage and I just re-read it this spring. The book gave me an understanding of what Alzheimer's is like from the patient's perspective. The book is funny, heart-wrenching, and recommended.

A Bit about Dad

Every story needs a villain and the disease of Alzheimer's filled that role. But a compelling story that provides growth and inspiration also has conflict. For my story, my father played that role.

Mom had just received the specialist's diagnosis of probable Alzheimer's. My father's first response was: "What about me?" I did not hear the bewilderment in those words. All I heard was the self-interest. He did not know how to look after my mother. It was her job to look after him. And while I would have wished for an integrated team approach, he was angry, frustrated, and bitter almost to the very end.

The doctors, nurses, community health workers, and dear friends all advocated that Mom be placed in care. Perhaps they could see that he could not cope but nor did they offer alternatives and support. I stood like a rock on the other side of the conflict. Mom would not be placed in care. I told him to leave, step aside, and I would do the job. But he stubbornly stayed, unwilling to abandon a responsibility he hated.

We constantly battled to find balance in the household. I hired staff so he could sleep and then eventually staff during the day to keep Mom safe from his verbal abuse. The staff was a revolving door and I learned that change would be a constant and that the perfect team did not exist.

Dad predeceased Mom by three years, spending his last six months in a nursing home. I was not able to give my father the same type of care, so I chose to care for my mother. Mom was agreeable and easy to help while Dad was argumentative and angry. Mom was my priority. I did my best for him within the nursing home, but I would not bring him home.

In Dad's last days, he was still angry and bewildered. When had old age snuck up on him? We did not speak much as our words had been harsh over the last nine years. My head was resting on his chest and his hand was resting on my head. And to my surprise, he gave me words to hold close: "We took good care of your mother." And "Why do we hurt those we love the most?"

On his passing, I chose words to process my grief. The first word was "forgiveness." That in death he forgave me for all that I was not and that I did the same for him. Eventually, that was too judgmental for me; the universe could take care of forgiveness. I settled on "acceptance." I was not the perfect daughter, and he was not the perfect father, but we did our best within our limited capacities.

I am writing this from a greater distance than the stories with Mom and I look for the reframe in our roles. I would never have had the opportunity to care for Mom in the way I did if he had been able to do the job. His inability gave me the opportunity to grow and love and develop as a human as much as the disease of Alzheimer's has. No one wants these challenges but they are what make us bigger and better as humans. Tragedy adds sweetness to life and can be embraced and even appreciated.

Sleep, Please Sleep!

For a week every fall, Mom would often come up to visit me in my home. Dad dutifully brought her halfway and we transferred Mom and I brought her to my home in the forest.

We were in high spirits and looking forward to some mother and daughter time. Unfortunately, since my last visit, Mom had changed yet again. She could not settle in a different place. She knew me but had never been to this strange place in the wilderness.

Night fell and I gave her sleeping medications, anticipating a good sleep. We were in the same room just in case she needed my help. Oh my, every half hour the entire night Mom was up. At 2:00 a.m., I gave up on sleep and we made blueberry jam. At 6:00 a.m., I begged her to just stay in bed for thirty minutes. I showed her the clock and pleaded for her to just stay there until both hands were on the top. So sweetly, "Of course, dear." Bing, up in five minutes. How she could function on no sleep was a mystery to me but whenever I make jam I think of Mom.

Managing Mom's sleep patterns so Dad could rest was the beginning of in-home care and locks on the doors.

Dad was so resistant to help but the lack of sleep was leaving him in a disgruntled and angry fog. Sleep deprivation for caregivers is worse than offering continuous care during the daylight hours. When we finally had care aides, the house had much-needed calm during the night.

Just Hug Me

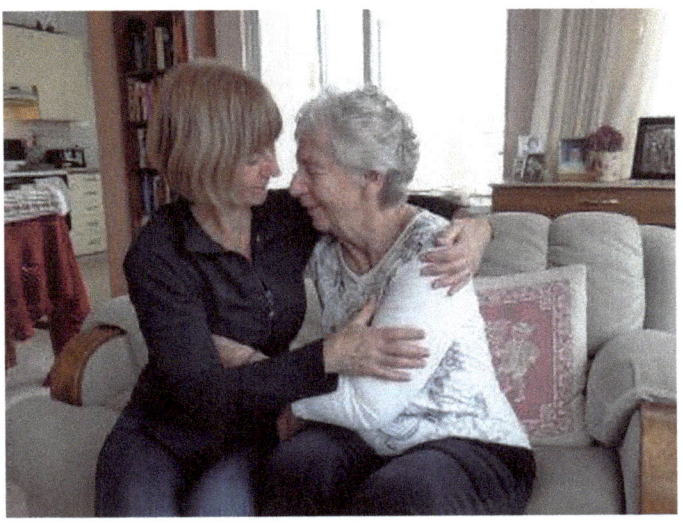

Mom and I sharing a hug.

live in the wilderness and despite putting stickers on the windows birds will smack into the window and fall hard onto the snow. Wings sprawled, twisted and helpless. In winter I rush out and collect them to keep them warm as the freezing temperature will kill them faster than their injuries. I have discovered that most will recover with a massive headache to join the flock later.

Cradled in my palm, I feel the bird's tiny heart beating madly. I wonder at the bird's fear of being clutched by a giant. Is this the end? Will I be eaten? Will my feathers be stuck in the corners of that massive mouth? And then the heartbeat slows and I know that the bird feels safe and sometimes even reluctant to leave me.

I wonder sometimes what Mom felt when she was confused and scared. And when we asked more questions she could not answer, perhaps all she needed was a hug and to be cradled in our arms.

Mom liked being touched so I specifically hired a team that would hug and massage her. I always felt that even though she did not know my name or how I was connected to her, she knew through my touch that I was someone special.

Saving Myself

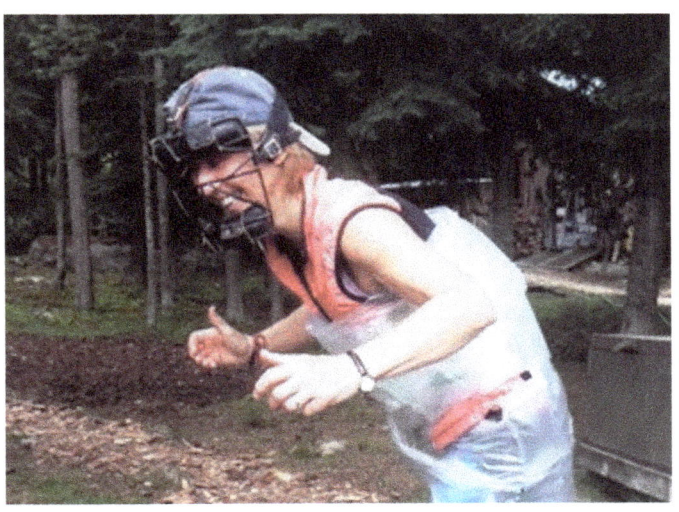

Safety head gear and bubble wrap for my run.

had no understanding of what I was getting into as the journey evolved. The beginning was just spending more time with Mom and taking her to specialist appointments five hours away in the city. As the disease progressed, it involved advocating and fighting my father for the best possible care for Mom. Later, it was team management and then finally palliative care.

Once I made Mom a priority and allowed the other things in my life to fall into second and third place, it was much easier. I also used acupuncture to relieve stress, I lived in nature and I ran. I ran my way through tears and anger and found peace every time on the other side.

I ran on trails in the forest surrounded by nature and this was very much an important part of remaining well. Of course, running on trails had risks. My husband thoughtfully purchased for me a back catcher mask to protect my teeth from the rocks and carefully wrapped me in bubble wrap. That final year, I fell hard four times. I like to think that if your knees look like a twelve-year-old's covered with Band Aids, you are still in the game! Still playing hard but in fact, my focus was pretty much shattered.

Somewhere along this journey my left eyelid developed a serious droop. I asked my optometrist what could have caused it and she replied, "How old are you? 55… hmm… Your boobs droop, your eyes droop. Nothing to worry about." I never noticed the condition as when I looked in the mirror my eyes are always wide open! It was my friends that pointed this out. It was worth heeding what they noticed about my stress responses.

The droopy eye worked out quite well as the other eye is a little more open than normal. The combination is not exactly what I would hope for but it has its benefits. When I face my husband with the droopy eye, it looks a wee bit sexy and sleepy, and is now my, "Come to bed honey" eye. The wide-open scary eye is "Take the damn garbage out!" In our marriage, communication has never been easier!

Constipation-Relief Recipes

I never dreamed I would be printing a "poop type" chart so that the team had a picture for a method of communication. "A big one" meant something different to everyone on the team and I do not want to go into details.

We tried teas, Metamucil, and laxative powders, and kept a detailed diary of this exciting process. Never had there been more discussion on this delicate subject. I also printed information sheets on high-fibre foods, and we stuffed Mom with raspberries!

In the end, these two recipes were a lifesaver. The fig whip could be spread on toast, added to yogurt, mixed in a smoothie, or just licked off a spoon. Mom loved to eat the cookies as did the team. I would make a big batch of everything and always have the freezer stocked. Cooking was a way that Mom showed

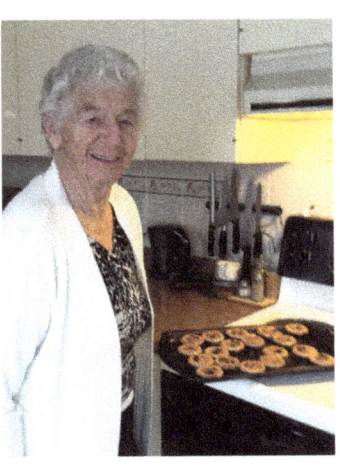

Mom baking fibre cookies.

us love and it has been passed along to everyone in our family!

Fig Whip: Beverley-Travis Natural Laxative Mixture
Ingredients: 1 cup each of raisins, pitted prunes, figs, dates, and currants, and 1 cup of prune juice concentrate. Check for random pits in the prunes and dates.

Directions:Combine all ingredients in a food processor or blender and blend until a thick jam. Store in the refrigerator. I liked to make a double batch in a food processor and fill sterilized 8-oz. jam jars and store those in the freezer.

Dose: 2 tablespoons twice a day. Increase or decrease the dose according to the consistency and frequency of bowel movement. Refer to that handy chart!

High-Fibre Cookies
Ingredients and method:
Beat 1 cup butter
Add ⅔ cup white sugar and 1 cup brown sugar
Add 3 eggs and 1 tbsp vanilla extract
Mix in large bowel 2 cups old fashioned rolled oats, ½ cup whole wheat flour, ½ cup all-purpose flour, 1 cup ground flaxseed (store leftover flaxseed in the fridge or freezer), 2 cups wheat bran, 2 tsp cinnamon, ½ tsp baking soda, ½ tsp baking powder, ½ tsp salt, and 2 cups raisins.

Add dry ingredients to butter, sugar, eggs, and vanilla. Mix just until even.

Scoop large spoonfuls onto a cookie sheet. Do not press. Bake at 350°F for about 10 mins. Pull out when still a bit moist. Over baking just makes these cookies dry. (I have switched out the raisins and cinnamon for dried cranberries, orange zest, and ginger. And the original recipe calls for chocolate chips. Yummy.)

Makes 36 large cookies each with approximately 3.9 grams of fibre per cookie.

Care Aide Angels Do Exist

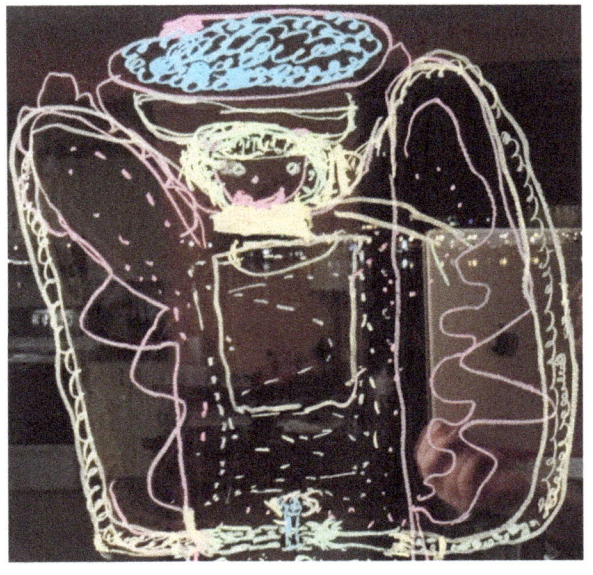

Angel drawing created by my sister.

had a care aide call and say Mom was mad at her and calling her Marlene and she did not correct her and was that okay? Hmmm, I guess.

After Dad died, it was easier but I no longer had a watchdog. More changes, more problems, and finally for the last three years of Mom's life, a team of angels that were more sisters than employees, de facto daughters or close friends for my mother. It was the family I chose that helped Mom and me through the last three years.

They found activities for Mom that kept her mind active and pushed the disease to the back corners of her brain. They researched the best foods for brain health and fed her from their gardens. They chose the music that she loved to listen to. They laughed and sang and read great books together. They brought their husbands, sons, and male friends around the house to flirt with Mom and oh did she enjoy that attention. My favourite prince of a husband fixed and altered the house to make life easier for Mom and the team. They took ownership as de facto daughters and did their very best for my mother. Some of my team did not or would not have the opportunity to do this for their mothers and they embraced my mom as their own.

And I shared. Not always willingly but with gratitude. It was hard to find that team. My father made it even harder as it was more about himself than Mom. But ultimately, even the short-lived care aides added variety to Mom's life and kept her brain active. I still see her gentle patting my father's knee and saying, "Oh dear, more new friends. I guess we will manage."

Bathing Challenges

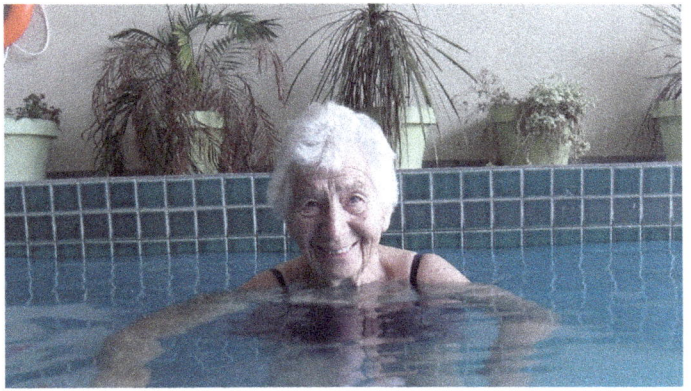

Enjoying a swim at the local pool.

This is one thing I think I did wrong. This is where I clung to my memories of my mother and refused to open my mind to other ideas. Mom loved the water, she loved to swim, and she loved to shower.

I still took her swimming as did some of my care team both in the lake and in a pool. She would swim the breaststroke, and I would nervously watch stroke after stroke, her face in the water not lifting her head to breathe! Yikes!! Finally, she would lift her face, beaming. It felt so good to swim.

As the disease progressed, she no longer felt safe in the lake. Perhaps she could not see well enough? Pool decks were slippery and change rooms cool and then eventually she hated to shower.

We bought a shower chair so she could sit. We bought a shower bench with a sliding seat. We had a big chunk of the tub cut out so she did not have to lift her legs to get in. We ripped out the tub and made a beautiful tile bathroom with safety bars, and we purchased a shower chair that could be rolled into the shower.

I asked her why she did not like to shower, and she did say it was a loss of ability that she mourned more than a loss of privacy. We covered her with towels for dignity and rubber slippers for security, and had a heater that turned the bathroom into a tropical zone. My team would be drenched with sweat by the time Mom was washed and dried.

And she hated it. Some days she was fine but other days she would cry and plead. And always she was exhausted. I had a professional care aide come to help with bathing as she had such confidence and speed it made the chore a little less arduous for Mom and the team.

In retrospect, it was me that could not see another way. Mom was not a stinky, sweaty old lady. Yes, she needed a good shower from time to time but for most days a sponge bath with loving hands would have worked just fine, giving her skin the care it needed, refreshing her body so she felt good, and not traumatizing her with what used to be. Forgive me. I did my best.

Hospital Stays

Mom had other problems beyond Alzheimer's and needed multiple surgeries on leg arteries. One of our cousins thought it would be handy if she lost a foot because then we would not have to worry about her wandering. That is black humour!

Hospitals scared Mom and anesthetic left her confused. She was sure she was being locked up. Our first hospital stay occurred without planning but subsequent stays went better. I could not leave Mom alone in the hospital if I did not want to return and see her tied to her bed.

The nurses were poorly trained regarding Alzheimer's and would speak loudly at Mom, telling her where the nurse alert button was, not realizing that she was not deaf nor would she remember the button. I was Mom's advocate, her voice, and I learned I could be powerful and effective if I kept calm. When I lowered my voice and spoke slowly, they took notice. If I stayed out of the nurse's way and did a good part of their job, I found that I was welcome in the hospital. One nurse even shared staff treats with me! Homemade Cranberry Bliss Bars that I can still taste.

But there was much I needed to find out for myself. A sheepskin costs about one hundred dollars and helps to prevent bedsores. So I bought one. There are better quality mattresses in the hospital so I asked for one. I hired staff to give me breaks but discovered the hospital can provide a sitter for free when you need a break. The sitters are not engaging but do keep patients safe while my staff had Mom laughing and flirting!

And while Mom was being entertained, I went shopping and looked for a shower. A trip to Winners got me a few items to wear as this was a surgery I had not expected. I felt it was wrong to use the patient shower in the hospital, and I was not going to check into a hotel for one hour unless I had a very handsome man with me. My best option was the youth hostel. I arrived with my plastic bag of clothes and cosmetics, and paid the princely sum of five dollars for a shower. I still wonder if they thought I was homeless and perhaps needed a hug.

At the hospital, there was a fridge I could put a little food in. A toaster and hot water for tea and coffee whenever we wanted. Warm blankets to keep Mom cozy.

One morning, I was sleeping on a gurney in the hallway when the morning coffee server made his rounds of the ward. I immediately begged for the first coffee, and as he finished his round, he stopped at the nurses' station and reported, "I have breakfast orders for everyone but the patient on the gurney." The charge nurse's eyes flew open wide. "What gurney? Where?" By then, I had rounded the corner in search of another cup of coffee. I mumbled, "No worries, daughter not patient.

More coffee. Please." The nurse sighed in relief. She had not lost a patient on the night shift!

On future stays, we booked a private room and I or a staff member slept on a gurney beside Mom. Music was a helpful distraction as Mom had never been a TV watcher.

One day, the nurse was treating Mom's wounds with a very harsh antiseptic. Mom screamed in pain. I looked at the nurse and asked, "Is this necessary?" If the answer was yes, Mom and I would suffer through the pain. The nurse said, "It is on the orders." Again, I said, "But is it necessary?" The nurse said she would ask the charge nurse. The wound specialist nurse came around and changed the orders to something less painful. I learned it was okay to challenge the treatment and ask for clarification.

Some drugs are easier on Alzheimer's brains than others. There is often a marked decline in brain function after anesthetic. I challenged an anesthesiologist and the hospital doctor. The anesthesiologist did his best to limit the depth of Mom's sedation and the length of time. The doctor's nurse backed me and the drug orders changed to a drug that impacts a brain with Alzheimer's less severally. It was a fine line I asked them to walk but with strong advocacy they did their best.

After a third surgery on the same leg, I asked the surgeon if he was good at what he did. The nerve! Bless his heart, he took that question as being fair. And took the time to explain he was pretty much as good as I could get and he was working with very old tissue that did not have elasticity. On one trip, the catheter had not been fitted properly and Mom was in serious confusion and discomfort. I did not want to go through that twice. The second time was no problem as everything had been fitted correctly. Something new learned.

And I learned it is good to politely check the drugs that are being prescribed. On the morning of our discharge, the nurse gave Mom a sleeping pill. We were not going to be going anywhere soon! That morning I should have asked for a review before any drugs were given.

I also learned that overall the nurses are amazing and it is the system that has flaws. Hospitals are unprepared for the number of patients with Alzheimer's and the staff is not yet properly trained. Mom had me so she was going to be okay. A hospital is full of many stories that are sad and hard. When I felt wrung out, I thought about the mothers with children in the hospital with no support and no money, and I sucked it up pretty damn fast. Mom and I were the lucky ones!

Best Car for Mobility Issues

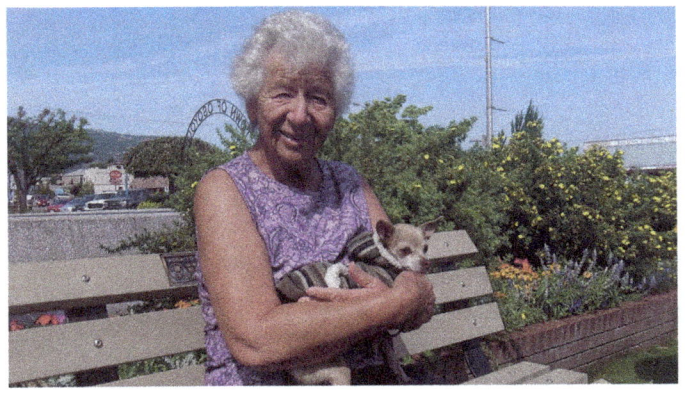

Enjoying a visit with a friendly dog.

Mom's team was driving an old Dodge Caravan that my brother had found after her car gave up the ghost. Lots of room for the wheelchair but it was getting harder for Mom to make the big step into the car. Plus, the car was acting up and I had fears that Mom would be stranded on the side of the road.

I need to back up. What was Mom doing that she needed a good car? Was she not locked safely in her home? After my dad died, Mom's life was full of activity. Every day, there were outings to the grocery store, the park, the beach, the museum, a cup of coffee and cake, and dancing! This was nine years into Alzheimer's and life was full!

I was confident buying a car would be easy! I would hop online and google "best cars for the handicapped" and find a list of amazing options. With an ageing population, this information had to be readily accessible. Car dealers had to be marketing directly to this group. When I checked, that was not so. Trips to the car lot with Mom would be required.

I hated doing this as when I was with Mom, I just wanted to visit with her and find fun stuff to do but I often was saddled with appointments and chores. Once we were driving from some appointment and I asked Mom if she still knew who I was. This was a question I seldom asked. She looked at me with her clear blues eyes and a small smirk on her face and said, "Sure I know. You're the one that is always organizing me!" Ouch. But there was so much truth in those words.

Back to car shopping. The salesmen would try and tell me all the amazing features of the car and took forever to understand that the ONLY important thing was getting in and out on the passenger side and fitting a wheelchair in the back. Who cares about mileage, warranty, and racy colours? Mom did not have a good warranty or low mileage and with her cataracts, the racy colours were lost on her.

I pre-shopped and then brought Mom to the dealer on the final selection to be sure we had the right fit. It was more like buying shoes than buying a car! You have never seen a person less interested in getting a new car. Are we done yet? Why are we driving in circles? Where was the stop for ice cream and coffee? What was wrong with the first car I got in and out of? Can't we go!

Finally, we selected a 2018 KIA Soul. A boxy little car with a big passenger door that Mom did not bump her head on. Close to the ground so she could get out with both feet on the ground and did not have to slide to reach the ground which aggravated her hips, but high enough that she was not pulling herself up and out of the car. Her depth perception was hit or miss and sometimes we had to place a bright-coloured piece of carpet on the ground so she could perceive the bottom of the endless pit that we were heartlessly asking her to step into. The seat was fairly square with a straight back. Bucket seats are just too hard to wiggle forward in. With a soft swivel or just a piece of drycleaner plastic, Mom could swing her legs in quite easily. Car problems solved!

At the time, little did I know that Mom would quit walking and dancing in just four months. The future was never possible to see.

Survival Techniques

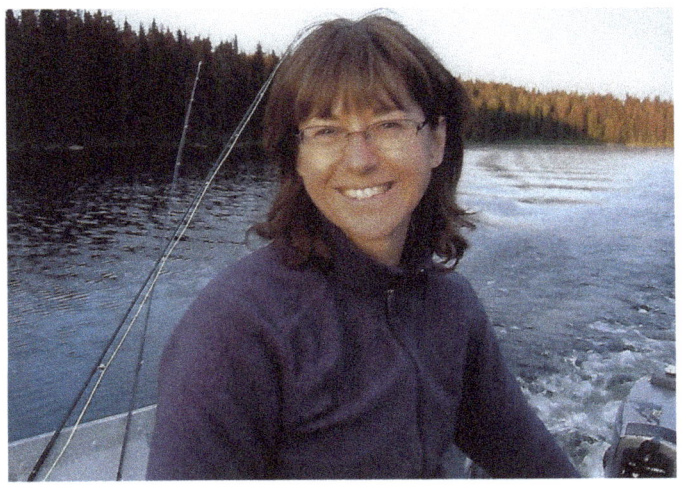

Heading out in the boat.

Nature is number one on my list. I have the good fortune to live in the midst of the wilderness and it never failed to refresh and renew me along this journey.

Exercise. I ran into my tears, I ran with my tears, and I ran through my tears coming home just a little bit stronger and ready to go on.

Building a team. There was no way I could do this alone. My team was the ladies I hired. They became friends and adopted family. They were with Mom more than I was and they loved her. Mom was the glue for the team.

Accepting that this was my journey and my priority gave me the right to do this first above everything else. My husband and my businesses fell well below the mark.

Acupuncture helped with emotional balancing.

Travel helped with mental balancing but over time travel became limited and was no longer an option as Mom was my priority.

Reading books on energy and motivation. Business books helped me more than self-help books as it is all the same message but presented in a way that worked for me. I liked Jon Gordon's *The Energy Bus,* and the One Word Challenge helped me with many tough times. My words in the last few years were "acceptance," "trust," "believe," "surrender," "laughter," "observe," "patience," and "gratitude." I would apply them to everyday situations and to the big stuff, and I always found benefit.

Meditation was one thing I could not do but I did learn to enjoy my first cup of coffee with attention and not let my squirrel brain start running for the first fifteen minutes of the day. Every little bit helps.

Whose Money Is It?

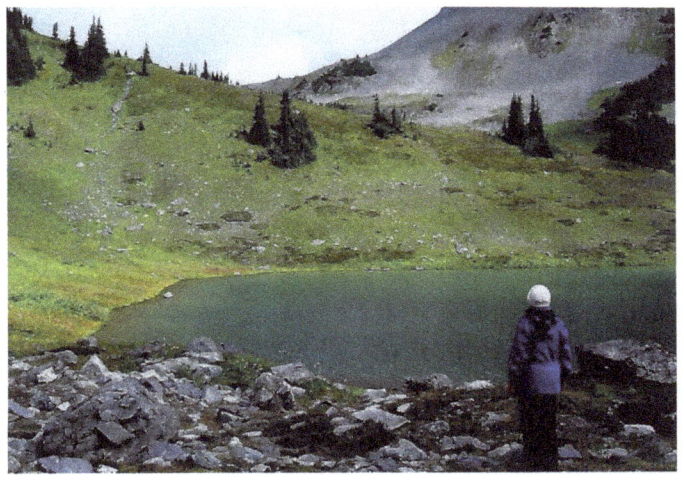

Mom out hiking.

Parenting parents was new for me. I never had children so this was a new experience. Money was a private, adult matter that was none of my concern, and I could not just tell them what to do, I had to ask. The thing with sending your parents to their room is, sooner or later, they come out and stomp their feet in a wobbly way and say, "Wait a minute! I own this house!" Finding that combination of being respectful and helpful is tough.

Looking after Mom while Dad was alive was difficult as he had always been a hard-working frugal man. Mom did the finances and Dad could barely read his financial statements. I simplified his accounts for peace of mind, but he was unable to make decisions regarding a reverse mortgage or equity loans.

The idea of putting a mortgage on the house he had owned for the last fifty years was beyond his thinking and well beyond my ability to convince him. I felt half the house value should be dedicated to Mom's care but that was a no-go!

Mom had a recent surgery and I used a very expensive care company until we could find our own team. I was away on business and just kept paying the bills without adding up the outflow. I still remember the feeling in my gut when I saw the total. I felt nauseous at the amount but even more panicked as to how I was going to continue this level of care. We needed a better approach.

After Dad passed, I was able to mortgage the house but the amount I could borrow was based on my financial situation, leaving me with limited borrowing capacity for my own needs. Had Mom lived longer, we would have had to sell the house or do a reverse mortgage to further pay for her care. The CSIL (Choices in Support for Community Living) Grant was the blessing that allowed me to care for Mom in her own home with ever-increasing needs. Mom always believed her home was her end-of-life nest egg and I had no concerns about cracking that golden egg.

There was lots I did not understand about home equity and reverse mortgages and bank lending in general, and the cost of care was well beyond my imagination. I should have talked to more than one money manager about the options well before we needed the funds. Thinking creatively and forming a plan would have saved my sanity and a few grey hairs and we would have had a little certainty as to what funds were available.

Possible Funding Options in Canada

The prevailing attitude was that I should step aside and let the professionals provide the care. I fought back hard against this thinking and found a better way for my mother. We each have to find our path but I was adamant that I would keep Mom out of a care home as long as possible.

There was a small pile of government money out there but it did require some digging. Shared stories from other caregivers brought me to our local community health nurse. It took a lot of patience but finally we received a grant that made a huge difference. There is nothing funny about money and I am forever grateful for the government grants I stumbled on to. For us, this grant became helpful for the last three years of Mom's life. The grant focused on funding for physical needs. It did not address or recognize the fact that Mom could not be left alone for her safety. But it did help with eating, dressing, and showers. Each task was measured and funded accordingly, escalating as the disability grew.

I could have also found this grant in an internet search for "Choice in supports for Independent Living" or "self-managed care programs in Canada." I flipped a lot of stones before I felt I had exhausted the options. A saying that helped was: "Never accept a no answer from someone that is not authorized to say yes."

The process to get the grant was not that difficult but very slow and Mom's needs were progressing rapidly. I did the bookkeeping myself and hired the team. We also added some of Mom's funds to the project of keeping her in her own home. I realize that I was lucky but also diligent in finding personal, family and government financial support for these last years of Mom's life.

Below are two important links that helped me find answers and options. The local community health nurse helped me with all the fine print and details.

Choice in Supports for Independent Living - Province of British Columbia (gov.bc.ca)

Help with Living at Home | Home & Community Care | IH (interiorhealth.ca)

The Dancing Queen Spreads Hope

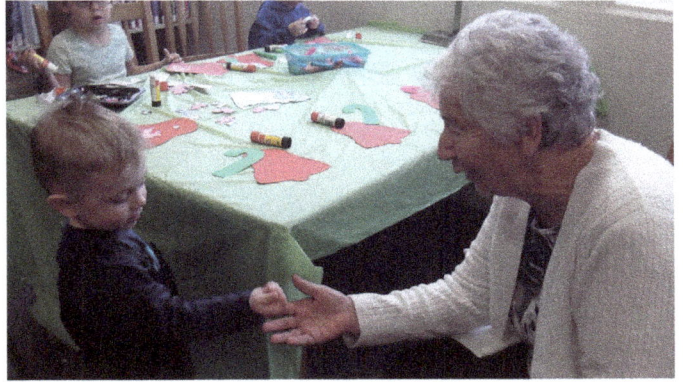

Mom at the toddler reading program.

The team was charged to find activities that Mom enjoyed. Every day had outings. Walks, the library, visits with friends, finding puppies to play with and children to hug.

One of the team took Mom to a toddler reading program at the library. At first, the program was not sure but as soon as they saw how the kids just loved having a grandma that dispensed hugs freely, they were on board.

Even asking if we knew of more available grandmas. The children would line up for hugs at the end of the hour.

Dancing had always been one of Mom's loves. She now danced three times a week, travelling to other communities to enjoy the senior centre's weekly dance party featuring live music. Mom would enter the hall with a yodel and everyone knew she was there. She no longer remembered the steps but would get up and circle the floor with her team member, shuffling her feet to the music as best she could. Occasionally, a gentleman would ask Mom to dance. Her eyes would twinkle with the attention and she would flirt a bit. Occasionally, a wife would get jealous! Sometimes the team member would have to fend off the focused attentions of a lonely elderly gent but it was all in the line of work.

Mom contributed so much to these dances as she brought hope and mitigated fear of a terrible illness. Many of the seniors were facing the beginning symptoms, some were caring for people with the disease, and here was an example of a woman clearly affected by the disease but still able to enjoy life. There was hope beyond the despair of the first diagnosis. There were options beyond the walls of a care home.

Window Shopping

was not prepared for the amount of involvement. Even though I did not live with Mom, she was always in my thoughts and I was almost daily solving a problem. It was hard for me to find information and support for the kind of care I was offering Mom. The medical establishment understands the cost to caregivers as being so high that the best course of action is to save the caregiver and leave the care to the experts.

I have just read a few stories about the emotional costs to caregivers when they place someone in a care home. Those stories reinforce that I did the right thing for Mom and me. Everyone must find their path and give at whatever level they can. I kept pushing the experts for information as they did have a lot of good ideas.

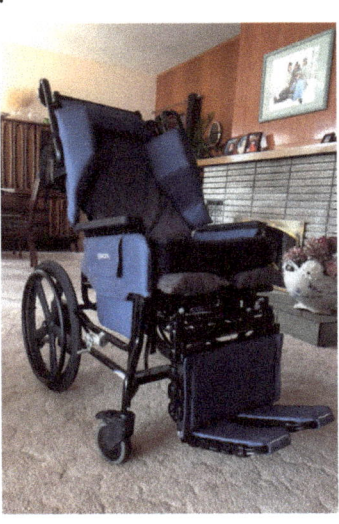

Mom's fancy ride.

I used to window shop for shoes and pretty sundresses, and suddenly, at fifty, I was excited about cutlery with fat colourful handles and really great incontinence products available in soft pink. My life had changed along with Mom's.

In a town close to Mom's I finally found a medical supply company that answered many of my questions. The internet was also helpful once I knew what I was looking for.

We bought fat-handled forks and knives, dishes that stick to the table, colourful and respectful neck scarves for eating. We found incontinence products that never leaked and skin-cleaning products that were very gentle. We tried mobility products like seat swivels, belt supports to help with lifting, walkers, and chairs of all types. Ultimately, we were the owners of a recliner that lifted Mom to standing and then later we owned a full-on chair to live in with a special seat cushion to avoid pressure sores. Special wedges for between knees and ankles made the final months in bed much more comfortable.

Mom was dressed in clothes to make dressing easier and shoes that fit on swollen feet but still gave stability. The adaptive clothing looks like regular clothes but has slits in the back for easy access. Most of the solutions are designed to give an extended quality of life and offer some dignity. My team loved dressing Mom in her new nighties and dresses with open backs. Mom always looked sweet and fresh.

In the back corner at the drug store, I found lots of helpful ideas like pill cutters and crushers. Elevated toilet seats and soft toilet seat rings. The hardware store carried grab bars that we had carefully and correctly installed. And the list goes on! Every problem I faced, someone had created a solution for at some time in the past. I just needed to look in the right place. It was a treasure hunt.

The Truth Is Not Always Necessary

There was a period where Mom would look for her babies. They had to be in the house someplace. After a family gathering, it was much worse for a few days. After the bigger gathering had left, I would stay a day or two longer to ease the transition.

There was a period where Mom was looking for her mother and father. She was so small and sad and lost we all wanted to jar her back to reality but that only added more grief. I asked her once how old she was when this sadness came upon her and she said, "I don't know. Maybe three?" That gave me the window to

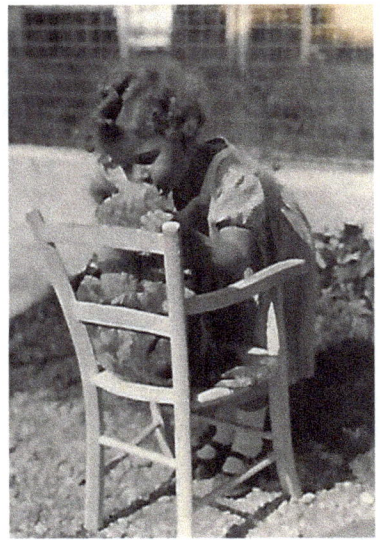

Mom as a little girl kissing her teddy.

understanding what I needed to say. From then on, Mom and Dad would be home soon, were on a trip or at the store. They would be back in a few hours or a few days and would bring her favourite ice cream. Whatever would buy me her smile. Telling the truth was not all that important.

But sometimes the truth is important.

Dad entered a nursing home a few months before he passed, and Mom would visit him there. She did not always remember who he was as her image of her husband was of a much younger man. Sometimes, she would have fairly elaborate suggestions of other things to do as visiting was not that much fun. We laughed at her ingenuity.

The day Dad passed, Mom and I sat with him for an hour. I did not know what she understood but felt I needed to offer her the opportunity to say goodbye at the end of a long marriage. We sat at the foot of his bed and she would peek around my shoulder at this man, now passed that had once been her husband. "Is he really gone?" "Ya, Mom, he is really gone." "Oh." "Is he really gone?" "Ya." "Oh."

Months later, we drove into the carport after an outing. I had just shut off the engine and we were still sitting in the car. Mom burst into a long string of random words and at the very end, crystal clear: "I still miss him you know!" "Ya, Mom. We all still miss him." Not hiding the truth was the right thing to do.

Mirrors and Reflections

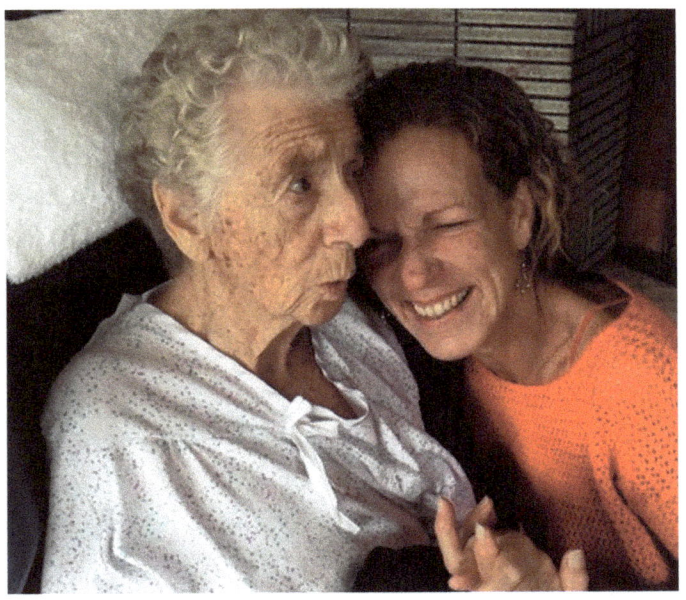

Mom enjoying a laugh with a team member.

Mirrors and reflections became a source of humour and concern.

Mom would greet the friendly older lady in the mirror and have a short visit with her. She would tell me what a warm smile she had. It made me feel good that she was not critical about what she looked like and still recognized the warmth in her personality if not the person. I would be looking over Mom's shoulder, but she was focused on the nice older lady.

Sometimes, I thought Mom was making a joke and knew this reflection was herself, but I have read too many other stories about this behaviour to believe that. One time, she lifted a heavy mirror of the wall and carried it into the living room to show us her new friend. Yikes! We all jumped before something happened. Changes needed to be made.

We covered some mirrors with posters, coloured wrapping paper, and scarves. The bathroom mirror was of real concern as Mom did not like being "watched" in the bathroom. This I covered with semi-transparent sticky paper with a frosted design. It worked great and looked good. Curtains were drawn at night to cover reflections in the windows.

It was sometimes difficult on an outing when Mom would stop to chat with her reflection but at least she liked herself! I am not so confident I would enjoy a conversation with my reflection.

The other benefit of having no mirrors in the house was I never looked better. The easiest way to remove wrinkles and lines is to take the mirrors away! This was the house I grew up in, so it was easy to pretend I still had the smooth skin of a fifteen-year-old. Once again, the truth is not always kind or necessary.

A Word about Nursing Homes

There is a prevailing attitude that once someone is in professional care you can relinquish the responsibility to the experts. I discovered that was not so and that I needed to continue to advocate for my dad when he was in a nursing home just as I had for my mother and husband when in hospital. I had to be involved for the care to be the best it can be.

My husband recently had surgery, and I would wait until the night nurse started her shift before heading home. The nurse came into his room and introduced herself. My husband informed her that I was waiting to see her so she understood he was not a homeless rubby. That somebody cared for him and would raise hell if he was not properly looked after. She gave him a critical look and said, "You don't look like a rubby—well, at least you don't smell like one!"

Advocacy is very important in any institutional settings. I had been sure that at some time I would be moving Mom to a nursing home but discovered that while it was a challenge at each new phase, I was able to adapt her care to provide for her in her own home. A team of angels was essential for this to work.

Dad was not so fortunate as he was not willing to let me help him and spent the last six months of his life in a nursing home. I often reminded myself that he made those choices himself and while I did not like them, they were his choices.

I did discover a few things to make him a bit more comfortable. After being admitted, he could still go home for visits, overnight stays, and holidays. He could go out for drives, coffee, or wheelchair walks. All visiting did not have to take place in the nursing home.

I hired visitors to keep my father company and bring him home-cooked meals. A medical consultant sat in on his monthly care-plan meeting to review his drugs and report to me. I provided a better-quality mattress. It was acceptable to leave a bottle of cognac with the nurses for a single shot nightcap (for Dad, not the nurses). Private physiotherapists visited three times a week to speed his recovery after a fall. I requested a pressure-sensitive mattress pad that would alert the nurse when he got up, helping to reduce falls. And there was a rubber mat to soften falls when they did happen.

Waiting to die is a slow process and the days are long. Most important, I discovered when there are no more words that would bring comfort sitting with my father; quietly holding hands was the best we could do and it was enough.

Trusting in the Good in Your Care Team

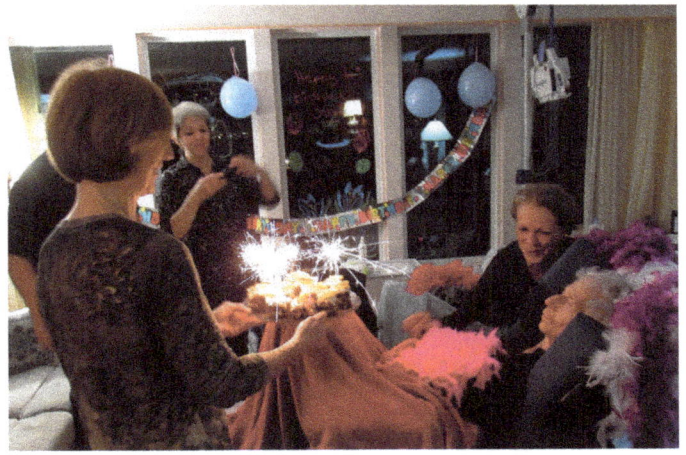

Celebrating another birthday.

lived five hours away from my mother's home and managed a team of six staff long-distance. The key-words were "trust" and "change."

I would just put together the perfect team, and there would be infighting over a toothpaste cap left off or a glass in the sink or crumbs on the counter. I hired a lovely person that had a difficult personality when working with others and took hours of my time in counselling and mediation. The daily logbook became a complaint book that was not patient centered. This was the most important part of my job and I was doing it poorly.

As Mom's disease progressed, I needed to put more and more care into the house. My father was also living in the house and unable to contain his frustration when dealing with Mom and unable to help me with the planning and care. Dad was an old-fashioned husband, so Mom was supposed to look after him. This was a role reversal he was not prepared for.

I hired women that dressed and conducted themselves inappropriately. I saw one care aide lean over and wrap my father's head in her breasts to give a good-night hug. He looked up at me from between her massive breasts with a silly grin on his face! One care aide did a "pop the balloon: birthday dance; fortunately, she was wearing clothes and the other gave him a gift of massage oil. What was he to think? He was enjoying all the attention, and life was improved for Mom, if still not great.

Dad was having too much fun with all the attention, and eventually, I had to take my father to a lawyer to have workplace harassment explained. The lawyer was kind and understanding and much to my surprise assured me this was not an unusual consult and if the behaviour was a deviation in character, it could be caused by a stroke or stress. So sweet to give me an out with my dismay over the whole situation. I hired better in the future. I was learning slowly!

The care aide that gave Dad the massage oil was also a staunch supporter of Mom to the point of removing my mother from my father's anger and having the police show up on her doorstep. She was 100 percent there for my mother, putting herself in the middle of high family drama. I also had my father fall in love with the sweetest care aide that managed him so gently, kindly, and appropriately but still was able to acknowledge that spark in an old man's heart. I am forever grateful to her for that bit of sweetness that she added to his life while he coped with his own ageing and the tragedy of Alzheimer's.

I hired a manager to manage on-site as I was too far away. And then I let her go. I created a logbook that was task and information specific. I did more and more training. I had a dress code. I avoided professional care aides as they were not able to offer the level of compassion I was looking for. And I never gave up and never quit trusting in the good in people. I hired people that were compassionate but lacked good judgment. I only hired one thief so certain drugs were monitored extra close.

I interviewed one woman that referred to my mother as an object and would not stop talking. She had a stern and sour face, and I knew immediately she would not be a new hire. Eventually, Dad took Mom's hand, and they snuck off to the bedroom. I spent another half hour trying to get the woman to leave. Finally, she was gone. I opened the bedroom door to find Mom and Dad sitting on the edge of the bed holding hands. They looked up at me and I was reminded of the scene from Mary Poppins: my parents were the Banks children. I prayed that Mary Poppins would show up soon!

Cataract Surgery at Eighty-Six

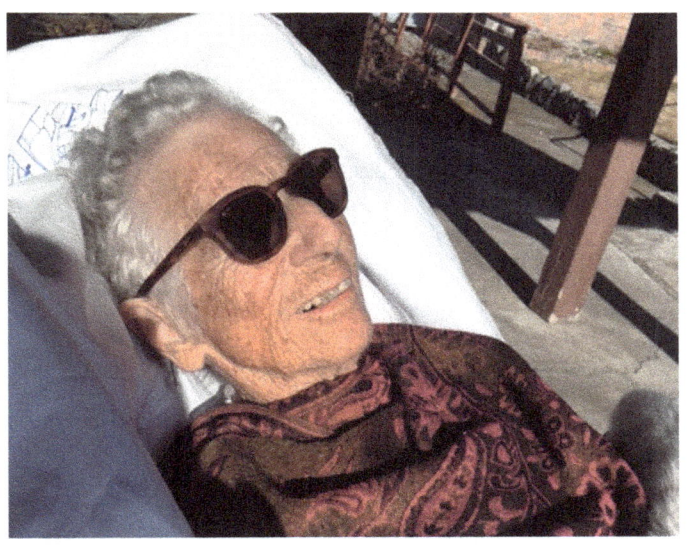

Mom enjoying the sun.

Mom's cataracts were slowly getting thicker, and her world was getting darker. Surgery would require anesthetic which was bad for her brain. The recovery required lots of drops and keeping her hands away from her eyes. And I had to make this health decision for her.

After the visit to the local surgeon, I tried wearing two pairs of sunglasses for a while to see how I felt. The brain adjusts to the reduced light but nothing is clear. Mom was still dancing and enjoying life but having more trouble seeing and feel anxious, so I opted for surgery. After an exhaustive search for a doctor that would not use too much or any general anesthetic, we booked an appointment for surgery at a private clinic in Vancouver. This gave me the option of choosing the time and date that fit best into my life as I was still working.

Mom did it! I was her coach. While in the surgery, her brain seemed to sharpen under the stress and she was gold. Angels guided the surgeon's hands. Whenever she wiggled, the tools were clear of her eye. We came out of surgery, and Mom was offered a snack and drink. Then the nurse looked at me and realized I was in much worse shape and quickly guided me to a chair before I toppled over.

And... after a complex regime of drops, Mom would not open her eyes for the next two months. I was devastated at having done the wrong thing and putting Mom through this trauma. We cajoled her and wheedled, trying to get her to open her eyes. Told stories of the spring flowers she was missing, the birds, puppies, and children. But nothing worked.

Then slowly her eyes started to open, and we were graced with their dazzling blue directness and kindness, and blessed with her smile as she could see us more clearly.

Sometimes, I did the wrong thing. Sometimes, I did what seemed to be the wrong thing and sometimes, it all turned out well in the end. Regardless of what I did and how it turned out, I was doing my best for Mom. The cataract surgery was one of the hardest things I did and I do not regret it as it showed me a capacity that I did not know I had. It would have been easier to say nothing could be done at her age and brain state, and let her continue to slide into darkness. It was not the easy road, and it still makes my stomach a bit queasy when I think about it, but it was the right path for Mom.

The Sound of Music

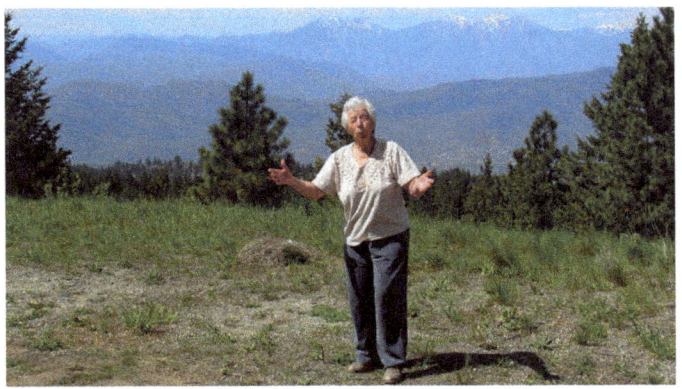

Mom yodeling and whistling in the hills.

There is lots of evidence to suggest when you can't reach someone to try music. Mom made the effort to reach out to us with music. There was the whistling year. She whistled from dawn till dusk. Drove Dad nuts until the day it stopped.

She would often direct the music with her index figure, smiling, always smiling. Maybe pausing long enough to yodel! Later, when whistling was no longer possible, she loved the André Rieu videos of Strauss waltzes. She loved going to the seniors' dance, and in general she loved the sound of music. A relative in Austria sent a few CDs of music from her childhood. The team would search songs on their iPads, and we all tried an online yodeling class! Mom was still influencing us in her final months.

Fresh air and music helped her through her last year. She was out in the garden the day before she passed, listening to Andrea Bocelli and Placido Domingo and feeling the spring sunshine on her face.

My Priority Shift

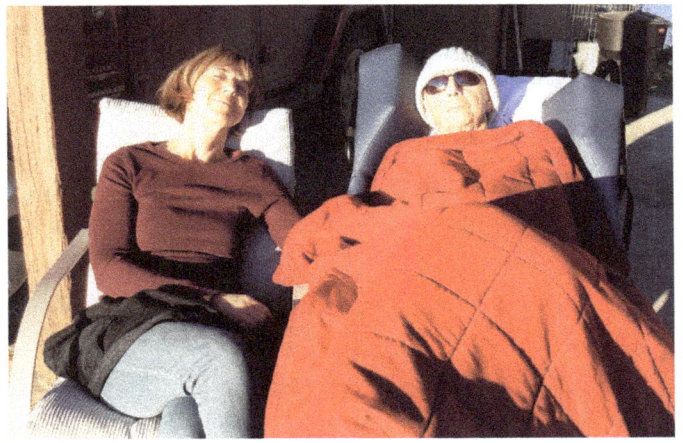

Mom and me enjoying the spring sunshine.

During the palliative stage, I learned that time was both finite and infinite at the same second.

A friend had given me a business book on procrastination called *Eat Your Frogs*. One chapter exercise was to quickly name the three things you had to do 100-percent correct right now! This was a business book, so they were looking for answers like, "Get my billing completed" or "Hire a new salesman" or "Execute an advertising plan." And there was an expectation to act.

I was past that stage in my life, so I was able to apply this principle to my personal life. The very first thing that popped into my brain was: "Care for my mother." Next came, "Care for my mental and physical health," and my dear husband came in third, my business was fourth. What was amazing was as soon as I was able to shift my priority to put Mom first, the rest of my busy life fell into place. I no longer tried to juggle everything into first place. Nine months later, my mom passed, I had survived the journey positively, and my husband and business survived in third and fourth place.

I am a busy person that runs full speed with a full plate yet that final spring I was able to sit with Mom under a beautiful red maple tree for over a month. If you had asked me three years ago if I had time for that, I would have said of course not, I am busy, and I have important things to do! I watched the tree go from bud to full leaf. I sat by her chair in the garden, holding hands, eating treats I had prepared for her, and I did not feel the rush of my life. This was the one thing I had to do 100 percent right.

Patient-Centered Care

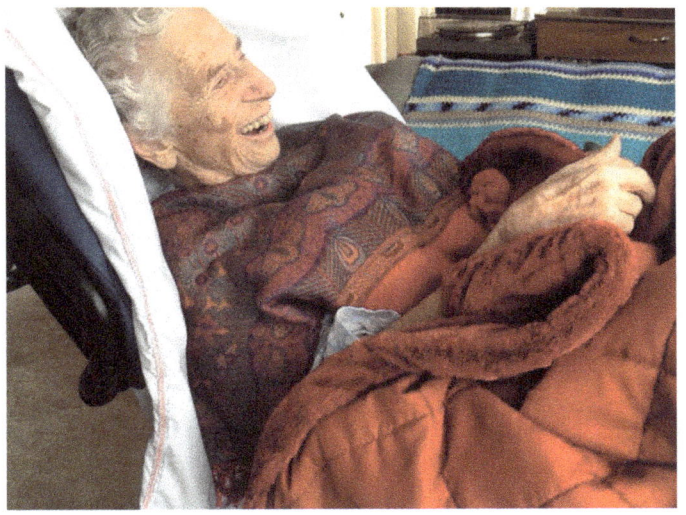

The team worked hard to create patient-centered care. It was all about Mom. When she could tell us what she liked, we would do our best to make it happen. When she could no longer tell us, we tried to guess and always respected the person she still was.

The team slowed down to a pace that Mom could handle on any given day. We tried to find activities that would engage her brain and keep her smiling. It was relatively easy as Mom was always a happy person who believed in finding the silver lining in everything. She did not love all the care aides but was generally kind and accommodating to their efforts. She did not love her physical and mental decline but made the best of what she had left to work with.

In her palliative stage, she still exuded happiness for the sunshine on her face and the music that was placed near her chair. We would open the front door and push her chair outside into the fresh air. She would take a deep breath and smile like a songbird coming out of a cage.

Her sense of touch and hearing still seemed to work quite well. And she could see and taste okay. These were the areas of activity we concentrated on. A bowl of ice cream, a local guitar player stopped by the house, a massage therapist twice a week, the warmth of sunshine.

Mom loved to read us *Winnie-the-Pooh* by A. A. Milne. I found this quote that sums up what we tried to do. Piglet asks, "How do you spell love?' and Pooh replies, "You don't spell it, you feel it."

Drugs and Humour

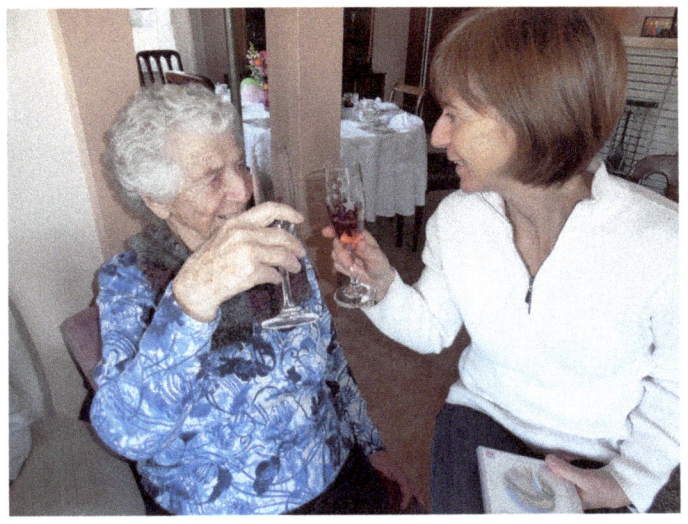

Mom and I sharing a bit of cheer!

The last year, during the palliative stage, when I was not with Mom, she was always on my mind. She was on very few drugs, but we were prepared for whatever happened.

We live in a small town so planning ahead was critical as access to drugs would be limited on the weekend. We were ready for whatever Mom might need. In the end, she needed very little and Mom passed easily, but until then, I could give people a chuckle.

They would ask how Mom was. I would say she was palliative and they would express their sympathy. I would reply, "No worries, it is not all bad. With Mom having Alzheimer's, it is hard for her to express how a drug might be affecting her. I have been sacrificing myself to test her drugs. A little CBD oil, a hint of morphine, a touch of Ativan with a top up of THC, and all chased with a glass of wine. It is all soooooooooooooo good."

Fortunately, I was not truly willing to try these drugs on myself, so Mom did have to soldier on alone. My drug of choice on this journey was exercise and nature, along with an amazing support team and my mother's incredible blue eyes that would see through me to my soul.

A Wet Issue: Incontinence

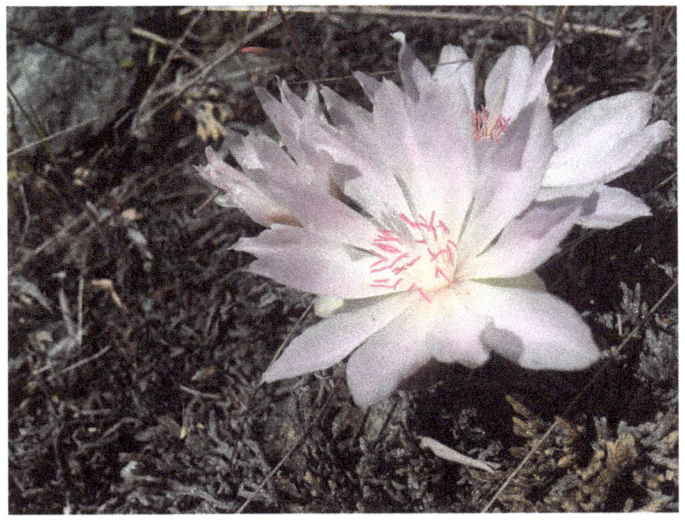

Mom loved rock roses and they do smell sweetly!

What I liked about caring for Mom at home was that it was all about Mom. We did not have to accommodate other patients or rules or even safety guidelines. We did have to constantly come up with new ideas and solutions—often, that was my job—like finding the right kind of incontinence products. It shouldn't have been so hard, but once again there is information that is not shared with those that are new to this game.

Caring for someone at home is counter to what our society thinks is the right thing to do. This set me on a path of conflict with my father, which was hard for both of us. At the end of his life, he ended up in an extended care facility for six months and he finally expressed his belief that we had done the right thing for Mom. I would have offered him the same care, but it was not possible. Once, I looked at him with love and said, "Do you know what your favourite word is?" His reply was a slightly puzzled: "No." And therein lay the problem for caring for Dad. He said no to everything while Mom would quietly and graciously accept.

Doctors and health-care professionals do not encourage what we did for Mom. Perhaps because they see the toll on the living as opposed to the benefits. Perhaps because they think with all their training they can do a better job than we can with buckets of love. And sometimes they are right, but not always.

Back to diapers. After months of the care team doing laundry daily and buying every brand of incontinence product that the local drugstore offered, I called a nursing home and asked what I needed to buy. I found a quality product at a specialty store that caters to serious medical conditions. A store that sold specialty chairs had way more supplies of much better quality than I found in the drug store.

During the palliative stage, the nurse was able to supply us incontinence products, which were a huge cost saving. But there was a constant frustration with my team as to how she would dole them out. Perhaps she had a limited supply or was convinced there was a black market for this higher-quality product. And she was right! I would have paid any amount of money to provide Mom and the team a product that worked, and avoid the frequent bed changes until we got the game figured out.

I also found mattress protectors, flat absorbent squares that took care of small leaks, very helpful. These I found at the drug store under products for bedwetting. Once we finally found the right products, Mom was snug and dry in the mornings, and slept much better.

Give Great Gifts to the Dying!

What was she waiting for? My husband said she was avoiding seeing her husband and her mother. My friends said she never had it so good. Six women that fawned over her, massaged her, and fed her big bowls of ice cream. A daughter visiting for extended periods. Life was never sweeter or more precious.

At this stage, she had forgotten how to walk and we used a lift to move her to a chair we could wheel outside into the sunshine. We would take her favourite music outside, and she enjoyed the warming sunshine of spring. She was squeezing the last little bit of sweetness that life had

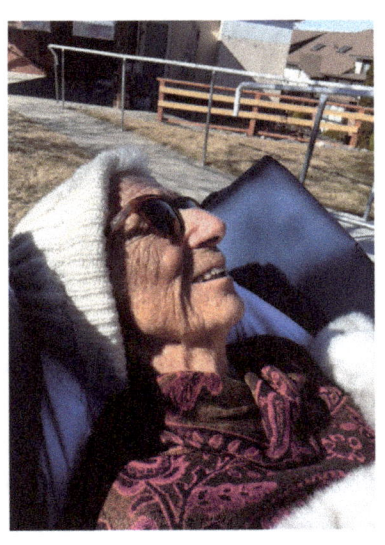

Mom with her new pricey sunglasses.

to offer. A whole basket of fresh raspberries, a dish of good ice cream, the touch of my hand.

Whenever I visited, I would give her my expensive sunglasses to wear when she was outside. For her eighty-seventh birthday, I carefully shopped for a three-hundred-dollar pair of sunglasses for Mom. I visited multiple stores to find the right frame—for Mom. I tried on multiple pairs to get the right fit—for Mom. The right style—for Mom. The right kind of lenses—for Mom. I worked with a care team of six, and I warned them that if these glasses got lost and someone was wearing them at the memorial, they would have some explaining to do! I learned that the best time to give extravagant gifts is when someone is palliative. Buy them the ring you always wanted, the best stereo for the music you love, as the odds of your getting those gifts back are pretty good! I now enjoy wearing that pair of sunglasses. Only used three months and I was heralded as the generous daughter. I think of Mom whenever I have them on. A win-win.

One of the hardest things I did was sign a medical scope of treatment order: do nothing to extend life. The paper sat on my desk making me feel that somehow I had failed my mother. That after all our struggles, all the problem-solving, I had failed. It was counter to every bone in my body, and as I wrote these words almost two years later, I immediately started to cry. Perhaps that feeling of failure still haunts me. Damn it. I did my best, but in the end, it was just not enough.

A week after I signed those papers, the nurse called to confirm my wishes as Mom had pneumonia. In a flat tone I said, "Do nothing." I hung up the phone thinking, *This is wrong.* We are raised to protect human life at all costs and even when it is "time," it isn't for those of us that have to make those decisions. I knew it was the right thing to do, that Mom would be okay with the decision, but my stomach churned for weeks. I decided to no longer extend Mom's life, but I also decided to make those finals days the very best they could be. Over the next nine months, that thinking guided all our care plans.

Wiping Mom's Bum

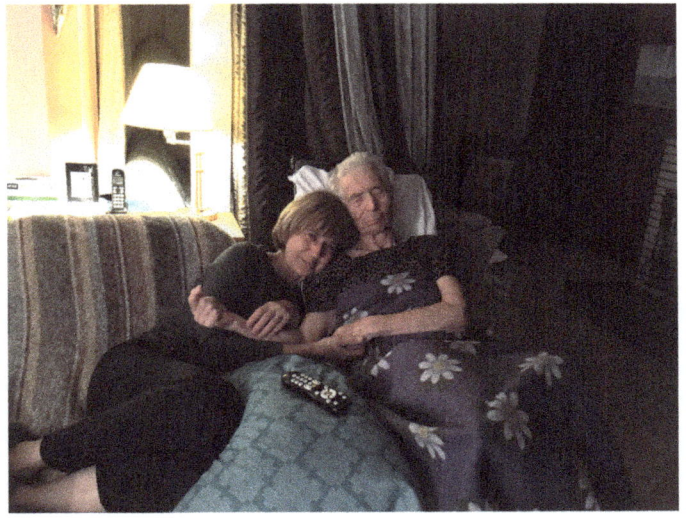

A bit of cuddle time.

I shared what I was doing for my mother with many people and they would say, "It is not your job to wipe your mother's bum. You shouldn't do that. You should always remain her daughter and not become her nurse." I couldn't have agreed more until I did it and then my perspective changed. They would look at me with disbelief when I said it was an honour to provide this small service to my mother.

When I visited Mom, I would let the night staff go and have the house to just Mom and myself. At this stage, she needed rolling over every three to four hours to prevent bedsores. We had been provided with an amazing mattress that was made of fingers of air. Sort of an egg carton of air tubes. Mom was the princess on the pea and was quite comfortable. But rolling was still required. Even the pressure between her knees was sufficient to cause a pressure sore as the circulation in her limbs was very limited.

I would set my alarm and, in the middle of the night, get up to tend to Mom. Romantic bedroom light just strong enough to see my task. Her eyes would flutter open as I disturbed her. Quietly, I would peak under her sheets and check to see if she needed changing. Always a happy, small excitement when bowel movements were healthy as so many systems had broken down. Armed with gloves, wet wipes, garbage can, and a fresh diaper, I would carefully change her. Our roles had been reversed. And while I am sure my legs flailed as a baby, hers did not.

When she was fresh and clean, I would snuggle her back in. Pillows and special bolsters carefully placed between her legs. Her skin was so smooth, and she smelled of baby powder and hand cream. Her curly white hair was soft. Her eyes appreciative of the care as they closed and she drifted back to sleep. There was nothing dirty or ugly about caring for someone at this level. It was simply what I wanted to do.

Flying From Bed to Chair

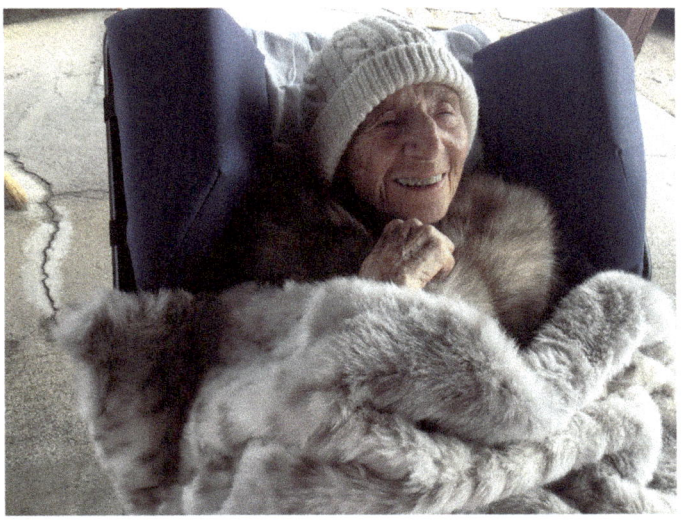

Mom out for a walk.

did not believe I could manage this entire journey at home. I thought in the last year Mom would go to a nursing home and my staff would go with her during the day, leaving the nursing home to take care of the night shift. It would all work out, somehow.

As each stage came along, I would learn something new. Sometimes the lessons came easily and sometimes the lessons were hard. I did learn that change would be a constant while caring for Mom. After dancing her way through year nine, ten, and eleven, Mom quit walking in her final year.

Mom still slept in her bedroom, and we had a variety of methods that were all bad for getting her out of bed and into her chair. I felt using a lift would terrify her when in fact it was me that was terrified of using a lift and of seeing our family home changed into a palliative-care home.

On my suggestion, my team tried to slide a board under her and then slid the board onto the flat chair and then remove the board and voila! So easy. Before this would be completed, Mom would be crying and the team would be crying and they would call me six hours away and I would be crying. After several weeks, I finally experienced it for myself and again we were all crying. The next day, I tripled Mom's drugs and she was laughing but that was not a good solution. She seemed fine with it. I need to also have the same dose of drugs for this to work!

I did the research and figured out a feasible plan, rented the lift, and purchased the hospital bed.

Mom loved the lift! She would swing like a queen as we gently lifted her into the air and over to her chair. One team member stuck flower stickers on the ceiling so her eyes had something to focus on when in bed, and at Christmas, we wrapped the lift in mini lights. With erasable felt pens we drew flowers on the living room windows to break up the grey of winter. The Christmas tree fit in the mini living room, and we had a lovely Christmas party.

I could have got a hospital bed for free from Red Cross. They have a lending service for many medical needs, but I did not discover that until after I had bought one. Palliative care eventually covered the cost of the lift. The lift company trained us on using the lift and helped with the installation. It was all doable once I wrapped my stubborn brain around this next change.

The Final Chapter

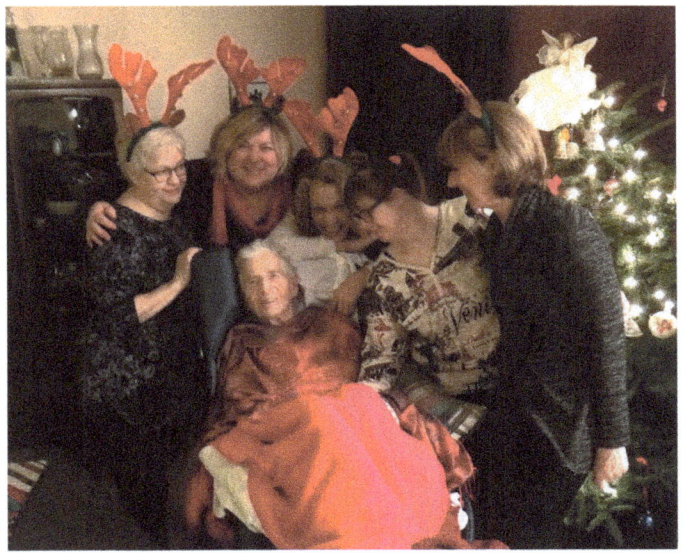

Cozy corner by the fireplace.

Mom lived for another nine months after being deemed palliative. At this stage, I thought I would have to put her in an institution but yet again, we found the path to keep her at home.

Her home transitioned to give her the best care. A hospital bed had been purchased and a lift rented. I started to move furniture around the home I had lived in as a child and then stopped as I could not go further. My head and heart were resistant to accepting this final phase and refused to help me do the work. With a heavy heart I went outside with a coffee to sit with Mom in the sun.

The team took charge, dragging furniture around and moving the bedroom to the living room. Curtains were hung to give her a sense of privacy, and we created a cozy corner by the fireplace with a sofa for visitors. Her new bedroom now had a huge view of the garden, sky, and hill, and was flooded with light. It was still home despite my fears.

With the lift and chair, we were able take Mom into the garden every day. The stronger team members were able to push her big wheelchair all over town. She loved the sense of motion and the movement of air on her face.

In the beginning, the doctors asked when I was going to give up and did not believe we could offer the level of care Mom needed. After a few months, they could see we were doing the best job possible anywhere and became supporters of our approach. I noticed I wrote "our approach." That was my care team, and I could not have been prouder of all of them. The Interior Health Palliative Care was also amazing.

Mom's house was a place of calm and laughter and love. Every time I came to visit, we had parties in the garden. We celebrated Thanksgiving with the team and then Christmas. We all wondered, *How long?* We celebrated Mom's eighty-seventh birthday in February.

Another great party with cake and a gift for Mom or the team (not sure which) of a robotic cat for her lap. Easter saw more silliness.

Eventually, other health issues were starting to take their toll. We were so careful, and Mom avoided bed sores with an amazing mattress pad, but we could not keep her arteries going without the "pump" of walking. Slowly her right foot started to die. The nurses bandaged and cared for it as best they could. Surprising to us, this did not cause her much pain as the nerves had thankfully died first. Mom loved to be touched, so we massaged her daily and I found the gentlest young man to give her professional massages when her muscles were all gone and she was truly just skin and bone. She would sink into his long, professional massage strokes and almost started to purr louder than the robotic cat. I was fortunate that Mom was truly the most patient patient.

It's Over

This was the biggest thing on my plate for many years and suddenly I had been fired, let go, made redundant. The team I built spun out into their own lives, and we made small efforts to touch base once a year. Mom was the glue, the true team leader, and I was her support. Not enough to hold a team together after the mission was completed.

We finished as a team with a final walk with Mom's chair, taking turns to ride in it. I visited Mom's house a few times in the following months and slowly prepared it for renters. We celebrated a memorial in fall with lots of family and lots of Mom's amazing recipes. We ate, we laughed, and we cried.

I gave myself time to adjust and truly felt I was

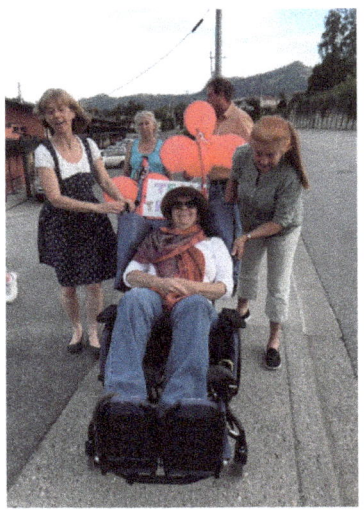

The team celebrating one last trip in Mom's chair.

doing well. Occasionally, for no reason, my eyes would leak for a moment and then my brain would switch to a mundane topic as though it knew I could only handle micro amounts of grief.

A year later, I was in the hospital with my husband for him to have a routine procedure. A tiny, white-haired elderly lady was pushed past me on a gurney. Suddenly, my eyes welled up and I could hardly breathe. I bolted from the hospital into the fresh air, totally overwhelmed by my response. Okay, so maybe I need a bit more time. Mom was no longer my priority, so perhaps for the next year I needed to make myself the priority. I had time for Mom, so I am sure I can find the time for myself!

Final Post

The end of my story. This was written just a few days after Mom had passed. As I read it now, I feel the same emotions.

Over the last few days, there are times when I feel I am in a movie script. The moments are so beautiful and poignant.

Thursday Clip One: I was holding my mom's hands from 4:00 a.m. to 6:00 a.m. Occasionally, both of us would sleep. There was nothing to indicate this was the last morning we would share. At 6:00 a.m. I gave her a little morphine as her breathing was a bit hard and then climbed into bed with her. I wrapped my arms around her, and we snuggled quietly as the day started to break.

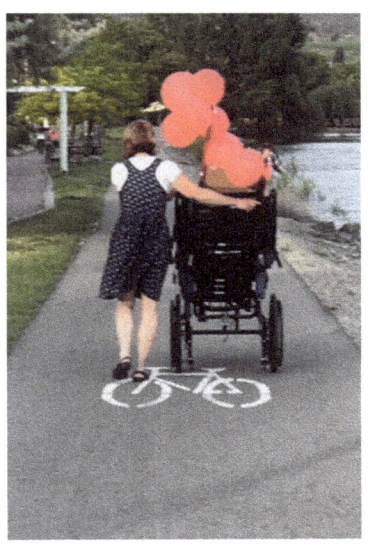

The sunlight was sneaking into the room,

and my thoughts had turned to what I would do for the day. Would Mom want to sit in the garden as she had the day before? Mom's breathing had settled. And then, while my thoughts were wandering but my arms around her, Mom slipped away.

I waited...there were two more small breaths. No struggle. Just a release from a body that was fragile and broken into a light that was pure and white. A quiet and gracious exit. I continued to hold her as my tears flowed. A team member was up making small early-morning noises. When she entered the room, I asked her to open the door to let Mom's spirit soar. It was so beautiful and just the ending I wanted, but I did not want it to end ever.

Thursday Clip Two: The funeral director arrived four hours later to remove Mom's body. By then, her care team had time to come and say goodbye. We washed her and dressed her in a blue dress. When they arrived, I placed a beautiful arrangement of flowers from a team member's garden on her chest. The stems were wrapped in a hand-painted placemat that I had made years ago. Mom was covered in a hand-knit blanket made by a granddaughter.

As I followed her out to the plain, silver minivan, I could only think that anyone receiving her would know how well loved she was. My parents always stood at the entrance and waved us down the drive. I did the same for Mom knowing that this was the end of a tradition of many, many years.

Friday Clip Three: My sister and I went to a lovely winery for dinner to celebrate Mom's passing. After dinner, we walked up a small bluff that looks over the small city where she lives. We sat on a bench and cried, we yodeled to Mom, we talked, and we hugged. She made a poem for Mom and recited it with her version of sign language. She gave me hugs that supported me to my core. And I gave her hugs that supported her to her core. We looked at the sky and sent our hearts to Mom. "M-O-M"—such few letters for the most important person in my life at this time.

Saturday Clip Four: I invited the care team, my rental sisters, and Mom's rental daughters to the house for a celebration of our journey. We put balloons on Mom's chair and a sign that said "TEAM MOM" and we took turns riding in the chair as the rest of the team pushed. We had to wear the expensive sunglasses, the beautiful pashmina shawl, and a cute sun hat. We laughed and looked at the world from Mom's perspective. The wheel-chair walks were one of her favourite activities in the last months of her life. We finished the evening on the balcony reminiscing on favourite Mom moments. On what she had taught us and on what we had learned. On what moment we would each hold closest to our heart.

Sunday Clip Five: One of our team members likes to go to church and although the rest of the team is not religious, we offered our support to her and attended a service that morning. It is a small congregation of a new ministry that is rather inclusive and Evangelical in some ways. That day must have been made for Mom as the regular service was shortened to make room for a very beautiful Southern bluegrass gospel band. A family of musicians with real talent and beautiful hearts. (Think of Dolly Parton's roots and you have the right music.) Mom loved music and was spiritual if not religious. Two songs were dedicated to her and sung by the youngest son, just twelve years old. Tears flowed.

Sunday Clip Six: I am home alone like an old dog sniffing around for a master that has passed. I have to make a list to get through the day. Make coffee, refresh flower arrangements, clean kitchen and tidy the bedroom, take balloons off the wheelchair, and call friends. Add breaks for unexpected emotions. All the things I did along this road to make it as good as I could for Mom. The coffee table changed to a soft ottoman to protect her from a fall, the first alarm system to protect her from wandering, the search for comfortable shoes, the adaptive clothing to give her dignity, the vinyl flowers stuck to the ceiling to give her something to look at and to keep her mind active and on, and on, and on. It is so weird that my mind no longer needs to solve Mom problems. So much time.

I looked after Mom for twelve years and would do the journey again. I learned so much and have such gratitude for the time we had. I thought that because I had done the work and seen the decline, I would be relieved that it is over. Sadly, that is not the case. But in time all will be well. I will surrender to the process and believe that this sadness will lift.

Thank you for allowing me to share my story. Mom loved to read us *Winnie-the-Pooh* by A. A. Milne so I will leave you with Pooh's words of encouragement:

If ever there is a tomorrow when we're not together…

There is something you must remember.

You are braver than you believe, stronger than you seem

And smarter than you think.

But the most important thing is, even if we are apart…

I'll always be with you.

Epilogue One

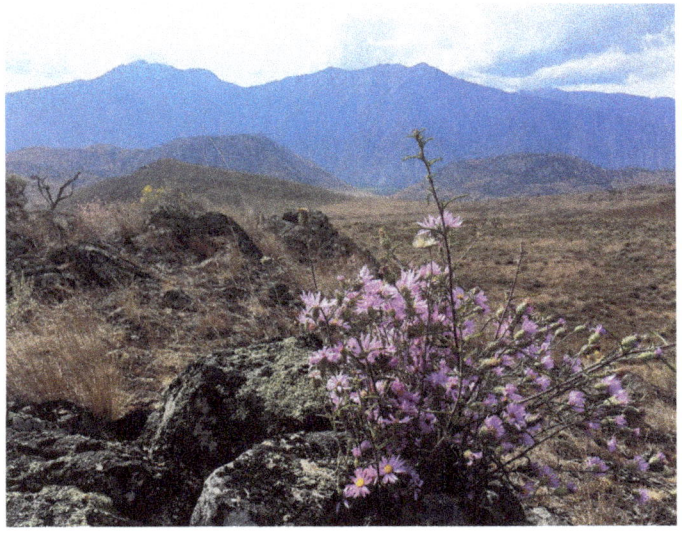

Mom's ashes were scattered with a view of the mountains.

t has been five years since Mom passed and I am doing great. As I prepare this manuscript, I shed a few tears and relive some happy moments and still feel the opportunity made me grow.

And... I wonder, at some time in the future, will I be in her shoes? Will I have the grace that she had? Will I be a patient patient? I fear that I will have more anger that my body betrayed me than gratitude for all my good years.

I am a person of action, so the best I can do for my mental health is fight back. To that end, I read books on health and longevity, I eat well, and I exercise. Maybe not enough, but everything I read points to movement as being critical for not just the health of your body but also the health of your brain.

And I made a vow to make lifelong learning a habit. I study Spanish, I am learning to sail, and I started alpine touring skiing and solo backpacking. And I have no intention of retiring from my work running a lodge. Some might say I am running from the clock and you can't stop time. But I plan on filling my time, however long it is, with a beautiful life full of adventures and laughter. Clint Eastwood was asked how he stays so vibrant at his age. He squinted at the interviewer and growled, "Don't let the old man in!" I used to walk to the end of the dock and dive into the water for a swim. Now I run to the end and fly like a twelve-year-old, looking down at my reflection. "Don't let the old lady in!"

Epilogue Two

My sister is starting to show signs of advancing dementia. I will remember that Winnie-the-Pooh thinks I am strong enough even when I do not feel it.

About the Author

Marlene Loney is the author of the blog Alzheimer's Blog Forum Canada. Inspired by the twelve years caregiving for her mother with Alzheimer's, Marlene recorded her experiences. She hopes by sharing these stories, she'll help others on their own journeys. *Laughter, Learning, and Gratitude on a Journey with Alzheimer's* is her first book. You can connect with her on the Alzheimer's Blog Forum Canada Facebook page or through her blog of the same name.